Imaging of Urinary Tract Diverticula

Vladimir M. Builov

Imaging of Urinary Tract Diverticula

Springer

Vladimir M. Builov
Department of X-Ray and MRI
RailWay Clinical Hospital
Yaroslavl
Russia

ISBN 978-3-319-05382-0 ISBN 978-3-319-05383-7 (eBook)
DOI 10.1007/978-3-319-05383-7
Springer Cham Heidelberg New York Dordrecht London

Library of Congress Control Number: 2014938363

Printed on acid-free paper

Springer is part of Springer Science+Business Media (www.springer.com)

To my family,
To my teachers,
To my patients

Preface

Urinary tract diverticula include pelvicalyceal diverticula (PSD), ureteral diverticula (UD), bladder diverticula (BD), and urethral diverticula (UTHD). Urinary tract diverticula are mainly congenital abnormalities, although they may also be acquired. In most cases the priority method for their diagnostics, especially if there are no clinical implications for a long time, is diagnostic imaging. Its algorithm, the same as most disciplines of radiological diagnostics in urology, includes, first of all, ultrasonography (USG) as well as X-ray and magnetic resonance diagnostics. Treatment methods for urinary tract diverticula vary from case monitoring to surgery which has been mostly endoscopic during the past decades. This monograph comprises a revised, modified, and amended text of *Diagnostic Imaging of Renal Diverticula*, a book issued in 2007, and rewritten chapters on UT, BD, and UTHD. The book sums up experience in ultrasonic, X-ray, and magnetic resonance diagnostics acquired from 1988 to 2013 in the urology clinic of Yaroslavl Medical Academy, namely, in "Avtodisel" Clinic Hospital, and in Railway Clinical Hospital at the Yaroslavl Station of the Russian Railways, JSC. We made a special attempt to provide our own observations as well as book data for all aspects of diagnostics of urinary tract diverticula in maximum detail in order to illustrate this study.

I would like to express *sincere gratitude to my dear colleagues* working in the abovementioned institutions, the specialists in ultrasonic and X-ray diagnostics and urologists of Yaroslavl and Moscow for their assistance and kind interest in this study. You are welcome to provide any opinions and especially critical comments on this book.

Yaroslavl, Russia Vladimir M. Builov

About the Author

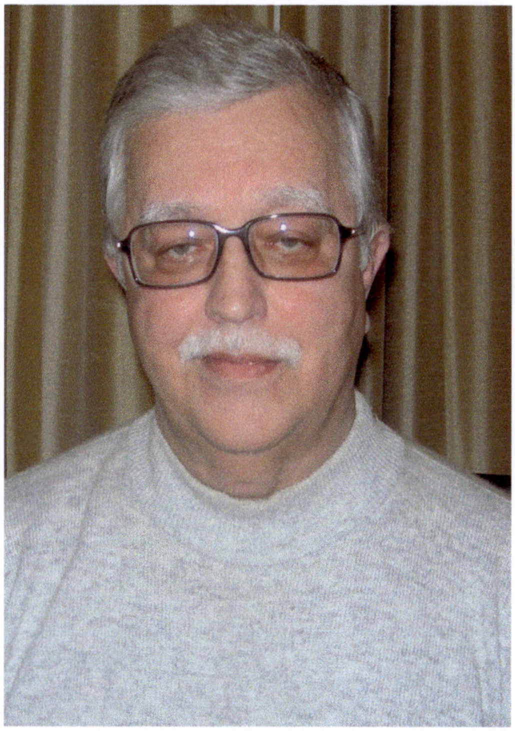

Vladimir M. Builov—MD, PhD, head of the Department of Radiology of Yaroslavl Railway Clinic of JSC "Russian Railways", and chief radiologist of the regional directorate of medical support of the Northern railway, branch of JSC "Russian Railways." He has been a member of the European Society of Radiology (ESR) since 1995 and the European Society of Urogenital Radiology (ESUR) since 1994. He is an author of more than 160 scientific papers on radiology published in Russia, Germany, France, Italy, Austria, and other countries, as well as 4 books on uroradiology. He is a chief coeditor of the *National Manual on Radiation Diagnostics and Therapy in Urology* (Moscow 2011).

This book covers all aspects of imaging of diverticula of the urinary tract, as well as issues of terminology, classification, statistics, etiology, pathogenesis, clinical aspects, and differential diagnosis. It is richly illustrated with ultrasound, X-ray, and magnetic resonance images. It is the first publication in the world that covers all aspects of radiological modalities of the diagnostics of the diverticula of the urinary tract. It is based on personal 25-year experience. This book includes the latest ESUR Guidelines on Safety of Contrast Media (version 8.1). The book is intended for specialists in radiology and urology and medical students.

Reviewer Valentin E. Sinitsyn—MD, PhD, professor, head of the course of radiology of the faculty of fundamental medicine of M.V. Lomonosov Moscow State University, head of radiology Department of Federal "Medical Rehabilitation Center," and president of the European Congress of Radiology (ECR 2014).

Abbreviations

BD	Bladder diverticulum
CAT	Computer-aided tomography
CL	Contact lithotripsy
CTU/SCTU/MSCTU	Computer/spiral/multislice urography
ESUR	European Society of Urogenital Radiology
EU	Excretory urography
LUT	Lower urinary tract
MDSCT	Multidetector spiral computer tomography
MRI/MRU	Magnetic resonance imaging/magnetic resonance urography
MSCT	Multislice spiral computer tomography
MU MCHCF	Medical unit, municipal clinical healthcare facility
NGHCF	Nongovernmental healthcare facility
PSD	Pelvicalyceal system diverticulum
RL	Remote lithotripsy
RMAPE	Russian Medical Academy of Postgraduate Education
SCT	Spiral computed tomography
UB	Urinary bladder
UD	Ureteral diverticulum
USDG	Ultrasound dopplerography
USG	Ultrasonography
UTHD	Urethral diverticulum
UUT	Upper urinary tract
VUR	Vesicoureteral reflux
XRCM	X-ray contrast medium
YSMA	Yaroslavl State Medical Academy

Contents

1 Diagnostics of Pelvicalyceal Diverticula

1.1 Terms, Classification, and Statistics

Diverticulum (di + verto) in Latin means a way to the side, a branch, and to divert and refers to outpouchings in walls of hollow organs such as intestines or esophagus. The same term is used in respect of the caudal part of the mesonephric duct (Wolffian duct) of embryos, which were the beginning of the ureter and renal pelvis

Renal calyx diverticulum was first discovered during autopsy in 1841 [1]. RCD or medullocalyceal dystopia (after M. Rauer) represents a small calyx with a much more peripheral location than the rest. Diverticulum duct 2–4 mm long and 1 mm wide is sometimes connected with the minor renal calyx and sometimes with the major renal calyx or, which is a much rarer case, with the kidney pelvis.

Until 1978 terminology for isolated cystous formations in renal calyces and pelvis included a number of various controversial terms. The following terms were used as descriptions for this type of cysts: *intrarenal cyst*; *peripelvic cyst*; *calyx cyst*; *calyx diverticulum*; *hydrocalyx*; *hydrocalycosis*; *pelvis diverticulum*; *pyelogenic cyst*; *pelvic cyst*; *pelvical*, *calyceal*, *pyelogenic*, *intramural cyst*; *localized obliterating pyelonephritis*; *calyx ectopia*; etc. The most commonly used terms were *calyceal cyst*, *hydrocalycosis*, and *pyelogenic cyst*.

A. Ya. Pytel and A.G. Pugachyov (1977) specified that "…cystous formations are located near pelvicalyceal system of the kidney, are directly connected with it or have a continuous or intermittent connection. The cyst can be: (1) connected with the minor calyx thus forming its *true diverticulum*, due to which many call such a cyst *calyceal diverticulum*, (2) located more distal in respect of the location of a prelum or occlusion of the minor calyx neck resulting from cicatrical process" (see Figs. 1.1 and 1.2).

In 1978, *calyx diverticulum* was approved as the official term by the Second All-Union Conference of Urologists (Kiev), and it was classified as a congenital abnormality, (see Section E for abnormalities of the pelvicalyceal system: (a) *pelvis aplasia*, (b) *calyx diverticulum*, (c) *pelvis cyst* [12–14]).

For the recent 20 years after the Second All-Union Conference of Urologists, as stated in the Urology Manual under the editorship of N.A. Lopatkin [15], a significant experience has been gained which required introduction of new doctrines into the existing classifications. However the proposed classification (1998), in our opinion, offers an unjustified reversion to the term *calyceal* and *pelvic cysts* which follows the term *parapelvic cysts* (move-after comma) instead of using the term *calyx diverticulum*. Such grouping has a wrong ground, since, as it is commonly known, parapelvic cysts come from lymph tubes of kidney hilum and are not connected with the pelvicalyceal system, while calyx diverticulum comes from the primary arteries. In addition, the term *calyx diverticulum* has been prevailing in foreign literature and many sources of domestic literature during recent years. An interesting fact is that unlike the terms *ureteral diverticulum*,

V.M. Builov, *Imaging of Urinary Tract Diverticula*,
DOI 10.1007/978-3-319-05383-7_1, © Springer International Publishing Switzerland 2014

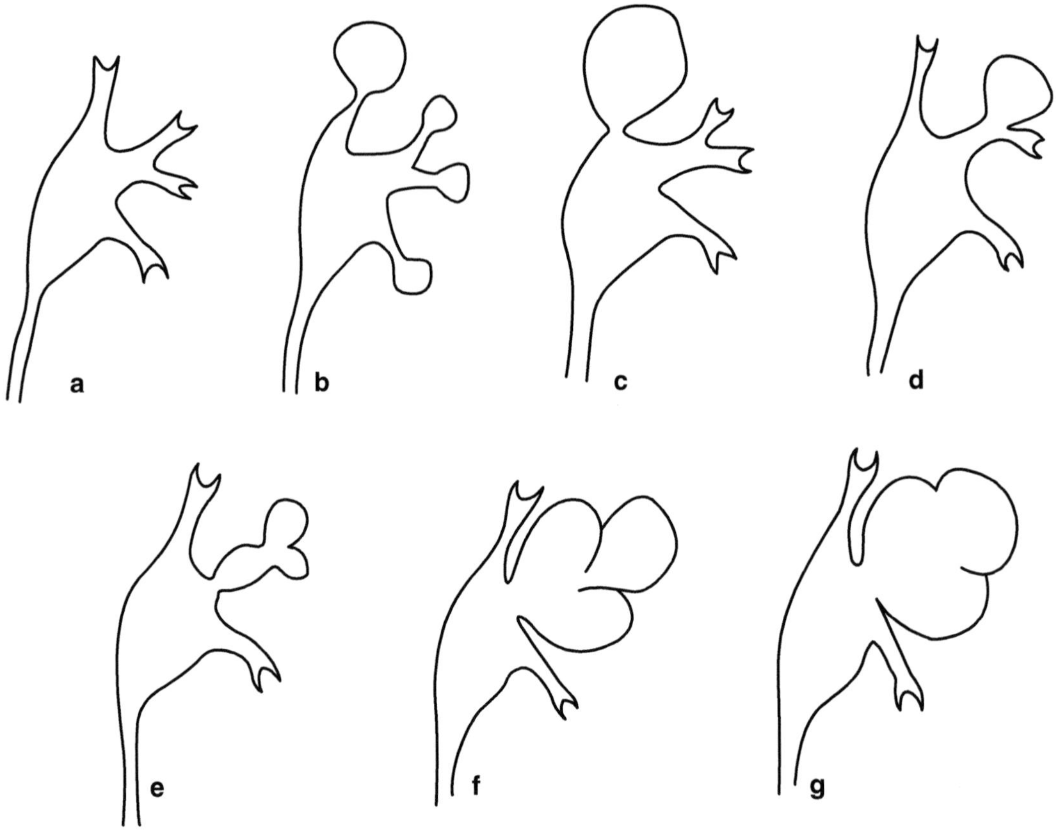

Fig. 1.1 Scheme of various arrangements of the calyceal cyst and hydronephrosis. (**a**) Norm; (**b**) hydrocalycosis of the forniceal and minor calyx; (**c**) hydrocalycosis of the major calyx; (**d**) hydrocalycosis of the minor calyx; (**e–g**) complex hydrocalycosis (After Pytel and Pugachyov [9])

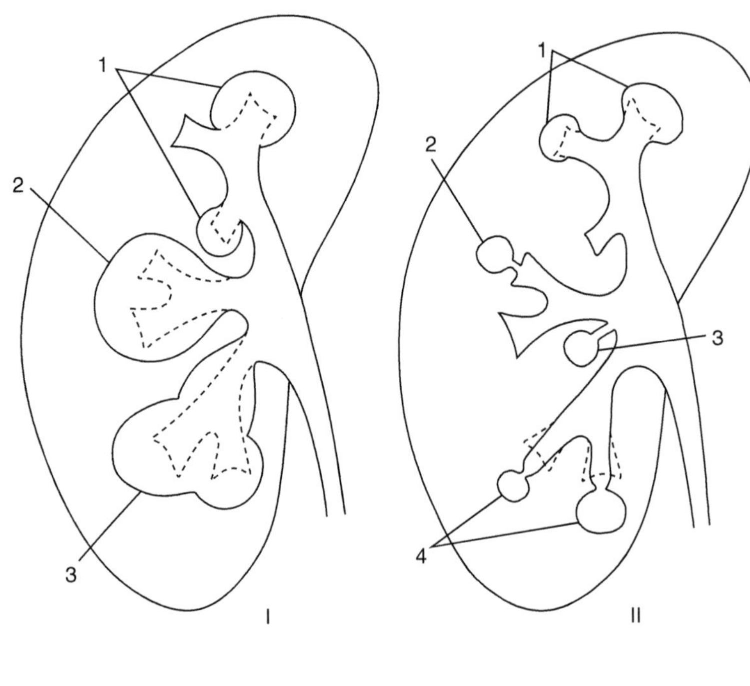

Fig. 1.2 Scheme of various types of hydrocalycosis and pyelogenic kidney cysts. (**a**) Various types of hydrocalycosis: *1* hydrocalyx of minor calyx; *2* hydrocalyx of major calyx; *3* diffuse hydrocalyx. (**b**) Various kinds of pyelogenic cysts: *1* forniceal hydrocalyx (Moore); *2* pyelogenic cyst connected by means of a duct with the minor calyx; *3* pyelogenic cyst connected by means of a duct with the kidney pelvis; *4* abnormality of the forniceal and calyceal area described by Dell'Adami and Borelli (After Pytel and Pytel (1966))

bladder diverticulum, and *urethral diverticulum*, which are commonly accepted and almost have no synonyms, the terms *calyx diverticulum* and *pelvis diverticulum* have got more and more commonly used only for the recent 10–15 years.

In some sources calyx diverticulum is called *Prater syndrome* (www.chelmed.ru/library/p.htm).

Up to 1955, 101 patients with calyx diverticulum had been described in the world literature.

By 1963 B. Abeshouse and G. Abeshouse had collected data about 318 clinical and 11 autopsy calyx diverticulum cases [4, 5].

By 1985 the world data had enhanced to 400 observations in 370 patients, including 103 calyx diverticula in 96 patients in domestic literature reported by V.M. Perelman and V.M. Builov [22].

At the same time by 1977, A.Ya. Pytel and A.G. Pugachyov had found descriptions of more than 800 cases of calyx diverticulum in the world literature [9].

Calyx diverticulum detection rate is the same in men and women and is 2.1–4.4 of 1,000 excretory urographies [8, 9]. In accordance with data by Middleton and Pfister (1974), pyelocalyceal cysts (calyx diverticula) are detected in 0.2 % cases in excretory urograms (quoted after A. Ya. Pytel, A. G. Pugachyov 1977, p. 74). Calyx diverticulum is found in children in 3 % of cases and in adults in 2.1–4.4 % of cases out of 1,000 excretory urograms examined (Wulfsohn M.A. 1980). In accordance with the data by V.M. Perelman and V. M. Builov [22], who published the first and the largest report in the domestic literature (52 patients with 53 diverticula detected), calyx diverticulum was discovered in 0.05 % of cases out of 12,000 excretory urograms.

Bilateral localization of calyx diverticula is found in 3 % of cases. Most often calyx diverticulum is unilateral. Calyx diverticulum is found two times more often in the right kidney than in the left one. Solitary calyx diverticulum occurs in 92 % of cases. Calyx diverticulum is found in an upper calyx in 67 % of cases, in a lower calyx in 20 % of cases, and in a middle calyx in 13 % of cases. Calyx diverticulum contains straw-colored liquid with urinary salts. It can be combined with some other renal abnormalities [9].

At the end of the past century and the beginning of the current century, the frequency of reporting of diagnostics and treatment of calyx diverticulum has increased significantly, and this abnormality of kidney structure can no longer be considered rare.

1.2 Etiology and Pathogenesis

Two anatomical forms of calyx diverticulum are known. In the outermost kidney segments, most often in the upper ones, small diverticula are formed with the diameter of 0.1 cm to several centimeters which are connected with the minor calyces. In the middle segment of the kidney, larger diverticula are found which are connected with the kidney pelvis or the middle calyx. Diverticulum cavity is covered with a secretory transitional cell epithelium; its walls may also contain muscular elements. Calyx diverticula are connected with the pelvicalyceal system by means of a narrow and short duct. Calyx diverticula appear on the 5–6th week of embryonal development when primary kidney artery spread branches toward the kidneys. Thus the main role in their etiology is assigned to local abnormalities of the renal artery formation. Abnormality of the arterial blood supply to kidneys is usually combined with reduction of collecting tubes leading to calyces of the forth order, which lose their ability to morphogenesis and expand under the pressure of urine [3–5]. During embryogenesis of the pelvicalyceal system, branches of the ureteral sprout normally degenerate and gradually disappear within the period of minor calyx fragmentation. In case this does not happen and one or several branches of minor calyces of the third or fourth order are preserved and then calyx diverticulum develops [9]. Among other congenital abnormalities, along with hydronephrosis and absence or hypoplasia of the right kidney, the literature contains references also to calyx cysts or diverticula as often accompanying inborn alcohol syndrome (http://history.km.ru/vsiachina/alconavt.htm).

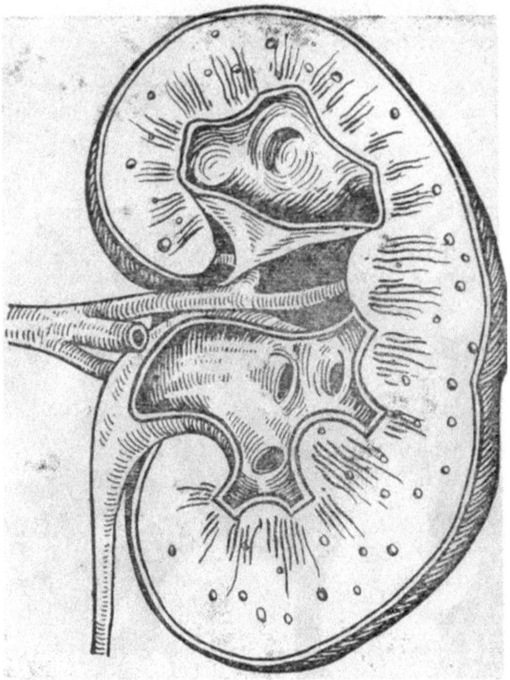

Fig. 1.3 Fraley syndrome, a vascular abnormality when arterial brunch is constricting the upper calyx neck which causes calyx cyst development (After Pytel and Pugachyov [9])

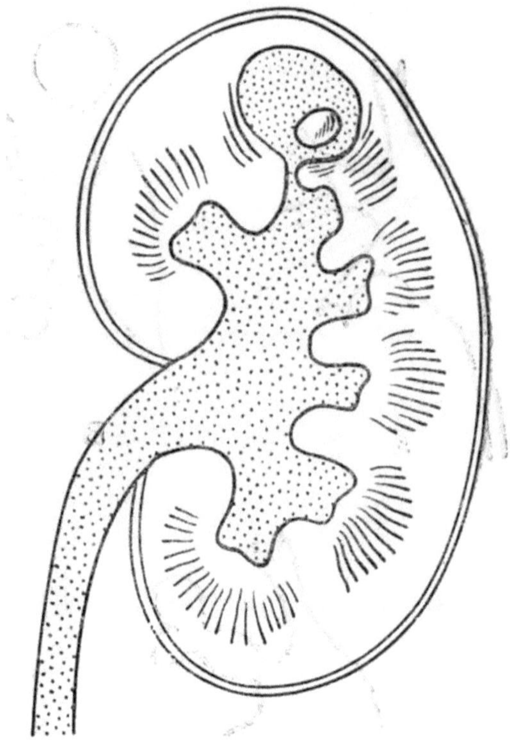

Fig. 1.4 A stone in a calyceal cyst (After Pytel and Pugachyov [9])

Some authors consider the possibility of acquired calyx diverticulum development. This happens when a small parenchyma abscess empties into the pelvicalyceal system, as a result of pyelotubular reflux and inflammatory stenosis of the minor calyx neck, as well as during hydrocalycoses caused by narrowing and even obliteration of the calyceal necks [6, 7]. According to A. Ya. Pytel and S.D. Goligorsky [3], a significant role in calyceal cyst and hydrocalycosis formation belongs to concomitant pedunculitis. When this condition is present, a tension of the abnormal vessel takes place which causes aggravation of loop occlusion of the calyceal neck; thus a calyceal cyst may appear due to constriction of the calyx neck with the abnormal intrarenal vessel, which is observed, for example, in case of Fraley syndrome [28, 29] (Fig. 1.3).

As well as A. Ya. Pytel and A. G. Pugachyov [9], we believe that the classification of this situation as calyx diverticulum is rather conventional, and it would be more logical and correct to address the development of obstruction in the area of the upper calyx neck as formation of local hydrocalycosis.

1.3 Clinical Diagnostics

In most cases clinical presentation is absent or defined by accompanying complications such as lithogenesis, inflammation, or spontaneous rupture [10–15].

Often an inflammatory process occurs in calyx diverticulum and an acute or chronic pyelonephritis, and in 38 % of cases stone formation takes place (Fig. 1.4).

The number of stones is usually not large (2–10) and they have a small size. There are described cases when up to 2,000 sand grains were found in the cyst (P. Rudstroem 1949—quoted after A. Ya. Pytel and A.G. Pugachyov 1977, p. 75).

When calyx diverticulum is infected or lithogenesis is in process inside it (Fig. 1.4), patients may suffer from dull pain in the lumbar region and sometimes from renal colic bouts. In accordance with the data by A. Ya. Pytel and A. G. Pugachyov [9], 15 % of patients have macrohematuria and 1/3 of patients have obstinate leukocyturia which is resistant to drug therapy. Cases of arterial hypertension are known among patients with calyx diverticulum which was complicated with pyelonephritis.

Upon examination of an overall radiogram of the urinary system, it can be seen that if radiopositive concrements are present in the calyx diverticulum cavity, they are usually located closer to the kidney cortex and may have faceted, polished outlines similar to structure of stones in the gall bladder (Fig. 1.22). If stones in the calyx cyst cavity are low in contrast or radionegative, USG and CAT can be helpful in their detection (Fig. 1.24).

Sometimes in the calyx diverticulum, cavity milk of calcium renal stone is found which is a mass of finest grains. Such a configuration is called *calcium milk* in the literature and is created by filling the calyx diverticulum cavity with a subtle colloidal fine suspension of calcium carbonate, calcium phosphate, calcium carbonate or oxalate, or calcium carbonate and triphosphate [38–41, 43]. Detection of this phenomenon, which produces no clinical presentations, is very important since it is often mistaken for a concrement in a calyx; thus remote lithotripsy and other respective therapies are used which are absolutely ineffective in this situation.

Some authors specify that calyx diverticulum can be caused by vesicoureteral reflux (Amar A.D. 1975) [27]. Among 32 children with calyx diverticulum, 23 were diagnosed with VUR. Calyx diverticula were different in sizes and were located in various kidney segments. In the opinion of Amar A.D. (1975), calyceal cysts development is to a great extent due to inflammatory process; 2/3 of young patients observed by him had signs of pyelonephritis. Thus when children are diagnosed with calyx diverticulum, they must also be examined to exclude VUR.

1.4 Ultrasound Diagnostics

As noted by A. N. Hitrova, V. V. Mitkov, and M. D. Mitkova, "Calyx or pelvis diverticula, pyelogenic cysts are almost never detected by ultrasonography" [44]. However, our experience proves that it is applicable only to small calyceal diverticula with the diameter less than 0.5 cm (Fig. 1.12) and does not refer to large calyceal diverticula (Figs. 1.13 and 1.16).

Ultrasound signs of calyx diverticulum, which were first described by us in 1993 [45–47], include:

1. Echo-free rounded structure with smooth outline which is located to the distal side of the calyceal fornix or the pelvis outline and is connected with them by means of a narrow passage.
2. The diameter of the structure is several mm to several cm.
3. In the case of *calcium milk* phenomenon, a combination of echo-free and echo-producing structures is detected in the cavity of diverticulum with a horizontal level which is moving during multiple-view scanning.

In the recent years, the so-called *twinking artifact* was described which had been observed at ultrasound dopplerography (USDG) of stones and calcium milk in the calyx diverticulum cavity which is detected in 91 % of patients. It represents hyperechoic structures with reverberation effect in the kidney parenchyma or a chaotic sequence of colored signals in the view of the stone or calcium milk, as well as along the acoustic shadow in the modes of color and energy Doppler mapping. At multiple views, USG and CAT scanning these structures demonstrate "gravity dependence of location of dense structures in the liquid formation" [48] (Figs. 1.5 and 1.21). Such a phenomenon, in our opinion, is similar to the so-called rattlebag syndrome described in radiological pulmonology when upon the patient's changing posture shifting of mycelium resulting from mycotic lesion of the sanitized lung cavities is discovered [44] (Fig. 1.5).

Pharmacosonography is a method which allows one to carry out differential diagnostics of liquid formations related to the pelvicalyceal system as well as of parapelvic cysts suggested by A. V. Amosov and G. M. Imnaishvilli in 1988 [50]. This method implies USG detection of expansion or absence of expansion of liquid formations against injection or intake of diuretics

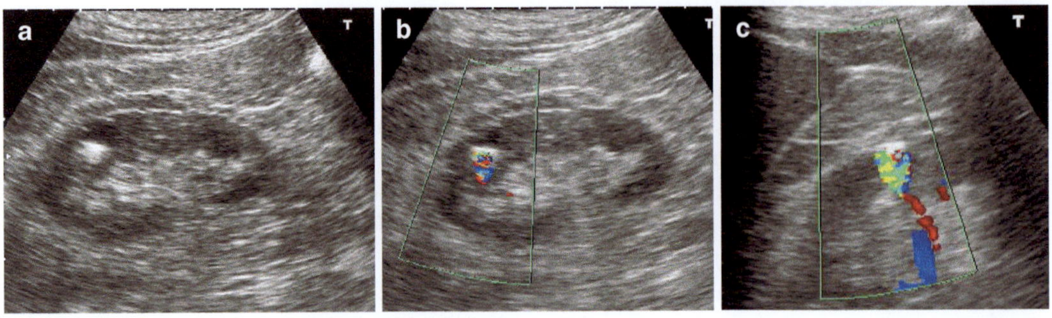

Fig. 1.5 Small diverticulum in an upper calyx of the right kidney with calcium milk symptom in sonograms and a color Doppler mapping image: (**a**, **b**) a small cavity with an echo-free and an echo-producing component separated with level line which shifts at turning in a sonogram of patient lying on the right side; (**c**) twinking artifact at color Doppler mapping (Observation by Gromov (2005), with author's permission)

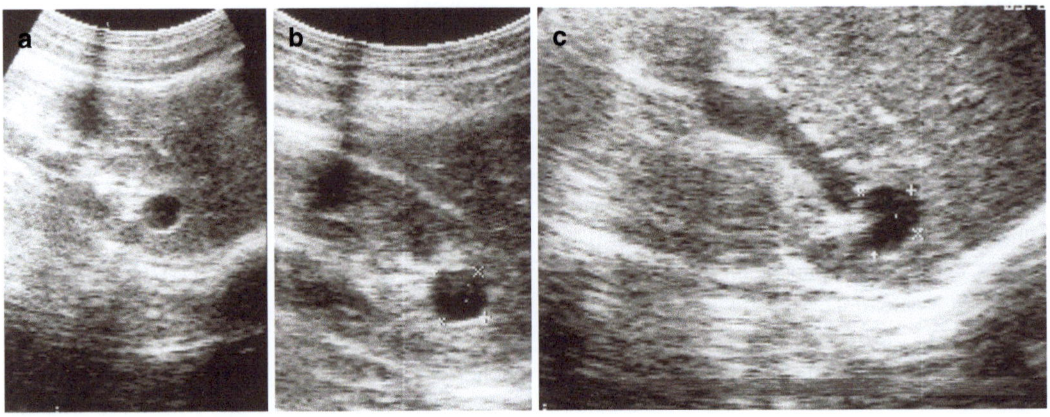

Fig. 1.6 (**a**–**c**) Pharmacosonography in case of diverticulum in an upper calyx of the right kidney (expansion of pelvis while expansion of calyx diverticulum is absent)

(Lasix (furosemide), bufenox). Thus expansion of a liquid formation proves its connection with the pelvicalyceal system (calyco-pyelectasis), while the absence of expansion may mean a parapelvic cyst or an intrarenal cyst [50, 51].

In the process of diagnostic differentiation of calyx diverticulum and isolated hydrocalycosis, a pharmacosonographic test reveals expansion of the ectatic calyx as opposed to the absence of expansion in a liquid formation resulting from calyx diverticulum, which cavity has a stable size during the test and becomes more intensive in delayed sonograms due to its retrograde opacification.

At the same time, it should be kept in mind that expansion of the liquid formation may be also absent due to pronounced expansion of the pelvicalyceal system when the reserve of the upper urinary tract has been spent (Fig. 1.6a–c).

1.5 X-Ray Diagnostics

The main method for calyx diverticulum diagnostics is excretory urography (EU), which, especially when combined with cineradiography and making multiple-view compression spot films, allows to obtain data on the length and width of calyx diverticulum neck as well as on other anatomical details.

In case kidney function is satisfactory, we believe that for the purpose of performing EU and investigation of the urographic phase during CAT with contrast enhancement, it is necessary to try to use nonionic contrast media for the majority of patients, such as nonionic monomers—Ultravist, Omnipaque 300, or Visipaque and others in the dose of 1.0 ml per kilo of body weight with the highest possible speed of intravenous injection. We deem that nonionic contrast preparations such as Ultravist, Omnipaque 300, and others and the only isoosmolar to blood nonionic dimeric contrast preparation Visipaque are the only option to use in all patients of the risk group (anamnesis including nephratopy, allergic reactions, diabetic nephropathy, congestive heart failure, use of nephrotoxic medications such as nonsteroidal anti-inflammatory drugs) In our opinion, usage of relatively less expensive 76 % intravenous ionic solutions of Hypaque or urographine must be limited as much as possible due to a much lower tolerance and higher rate and intensity of side reactions and complications. At the same time it should be kept in mind that in spite of a great progress in development of contrast preparations, even the newest of them require the medical personnel to know their usage procedures as well as possible reactions and complications, preventive measures, and treatment. All these issues are highlighted in the Contrast Media Guidelines developed by the European Society of Urogenital Radiology (ESUR) (see Supplement).

In excretory urograms, usually a small rounded shadow can be seen to the lateral side of the fornix of the minor calyx which is connected with the calyx by a small narrow channel. In urograms made later, the degree of contrast of calyx diverticulum cavity is increasing with emptying which in turn results in decrease of contrast intensity of pelvicalyceal systems (Fig. 1.18).

The survey radiograph looks specific in case there are so-called milk of calcium renal stones in the calyx diverticulum cavity (Garrett and Holland 1973). When calcium milk phenomenon is present, as it was mentioned above, the calyx diverticulum cavity is filled with a subtle colloidal fine suspension of calcium carbonate, calcium phosphate, calcium carbonate or oxalate, or calcium carbonate, and triphosphate [40–44]. Then an intensive boundary is defined in the X-ray image which shifts to the horizontal level when the patient turns (Figs. 1.26, 1.27, 1.28, 1.29, 1.30, 1.31, and 1.32).

In case of calyx diverticulum, it is recommended to have USG and EU tests with images taken in 1 and 3 h. From our point of view, a delayed image taken in the 30–45th min is enough, which depends on the calyx diverticulum size, the most common size being from several millimeters to several centimeters [41].

As can be concluded, calyx diverticulum has the following radiographic features:

1. A rounded cavity with smooth sharp outlines which is located to the distal side of the calyceal fornix or pelvis outline and is connected with them by a narrow passage which is often not visible in excretory urograms.
2. Calyx diverticulum cavity is several millimeters to several centimeters in diameter:– Calyx diverticulum contrast intensity increases in urograms made later, as opposed to decrease in pelvicalyceal system contrast intensity in delayed images.
3. Absence of motor activity of diverticulum walls as opposed to the walls of pelvicalyceal system which are detected by means of excretory cineradiographic calyceal-pelvic-ureteroscopy.

Spiral computed tomography and multislice computer tomography (SCT and MSCT) with image reconstruction in the urographic phase (SCTU) which appeared in the recent years allow to clarify calyx diverticulum anatomic details and define the density of concrements in accordance with the Hounsfield scale. This is especially important for choosing a method of treatment: remote lithotripsy (RL), endoscopic surgery with contact lithotripsy (CL), or conventional open surgery [21–29].

Thus application of USG and X-ray technique helps to obtain comprehensive information on the calyx diverticulum, its neck, presence of calcium milk, or a concrement in its cavity which is the principal factor in selection of a treatment method.

1.6 Magnetic Resonance Diagnostics (Magnetic Resonance Imaging and Urography)

The main method of upper urinary tract investigation along the whole of its length until the mid-1980s was X-ray technique with intravenous or retro- and antegrade introduction of iodinated contrast agent. The first reports on a possibility of making images of the upper urinary tract without introduction of iodinated contrast media at MRI, the so-called magnetic resonance urography method, using T2-weighted images in the frontal projection and the mode of suppression of signals from fat appeared in 1986 (Henning J. et al.). In our country, the first reference to clinical usage of MRU was made by Yu. N. Belenkov, O. I. Belichenko, V. E. Sinitsin, and M. Ch. Tavzadze [58, 59]. Invention of MRU technology is compared by many authors with invention of EU in respect of its significance for diagnostics of urological diseases. Apart from the possibility to visualize the upper urinary tract while avoiding introduction of contrast media and exposure of patients to radiation, MRU has become the first method which allowed to implement a 3D reconstruction of an image, rotation of an image in any plane with selection of the best projection, as well as the function of virtual endoscopy of the upper urinary tract [60].

MRU method principle is the following: When MRI is being carried out in the hydrographic mode, a highly intensive MR signal is registered which comes from stationary or quasi-stationary liquid located in natural or pathological structures against the background of a much less intensive signal from surrounding organs and tissues. This helps to obtain sharp images of urinary tract, especially in case it is expanded. In order to improve images, especially those of unexpanded urinary tract and smaller calyx diverticula, methods based on using loop diuretics were suggested (Lasix (furosemide)). They are introduced parenterally prior to MRU, which provide a quick diuretic effect and causes expansion of pelvicalyceal systems and ureters which improves their visualization. In addition to intravenous introduction of furosemide, also external compression of ureters was suggested. However for the best visualization of urinary tract, introduction of paramagnetic contrast materials is required, including cases of combination with diuretic load [59–63] (Figs. 1.7, 1.8, and 1.9).

Thus MRU is becoming the most perspective method for examination of the upper urinary tract, especially in children and in those cases when usage of roentgenocontrast preparations for

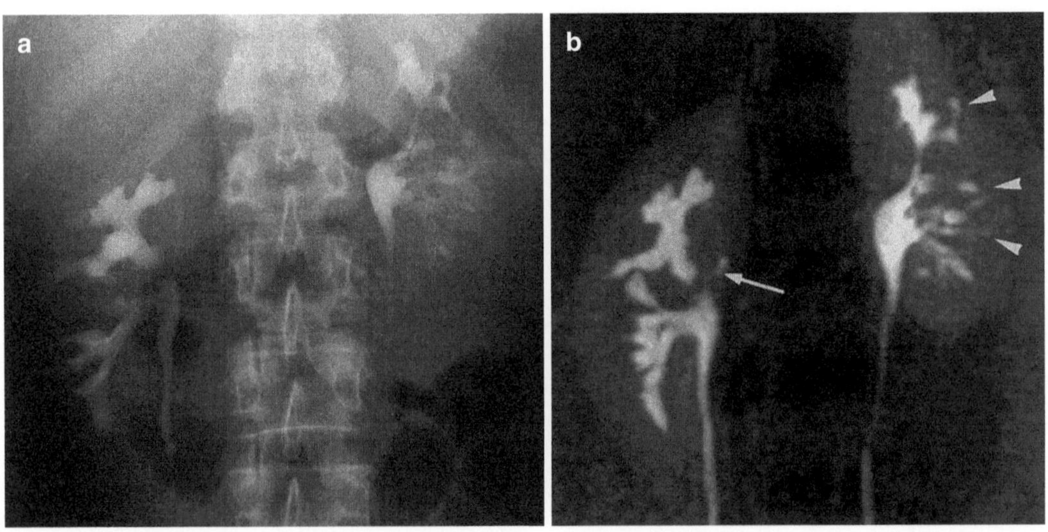

Fig. 1.7 (**a**) A small diverticulum in the right kidney pelvis cannot be seen in the excretory urogram; (**b**) the same diverticulum diverticula (*arrow*-in the right and *arrow-head* in the left kidneys) can be well distinguished in the magnetic resonance urogram (Nolte-Ernsting et al. [59])

EU is not possible or not recommended. The only drawback of MRU, which is, unfortunately, significant and difficult to overcome in many countries, is the high cost of magnetic resonance imaging units and paramagnetic contrast media. In major works issued in Russia by V.I. Dombrovsky [57] and Yu. G. Alyaev, V.E. Sinitsyn, and N. A. Grigoriev (2005) which are devoted to MRI in urology, their high efficiency and superiority over other kinds of diagnostics is highlighted. At the same time it is specified that these systems are still rather few; that is why "MRI usually serves as "second-tier" diagnostics to clarify data from preceding tests." Thanks to implementation of the health investment program, the number of MRI systems has been constantly growing in our country during the recent years; therefore 2010 algorithm in urological radiology is optimal in our opinion, provided modern modifications of USG and MRI are used. The latter, which used to be a "second-tier" diagnostic method [56], considering data from

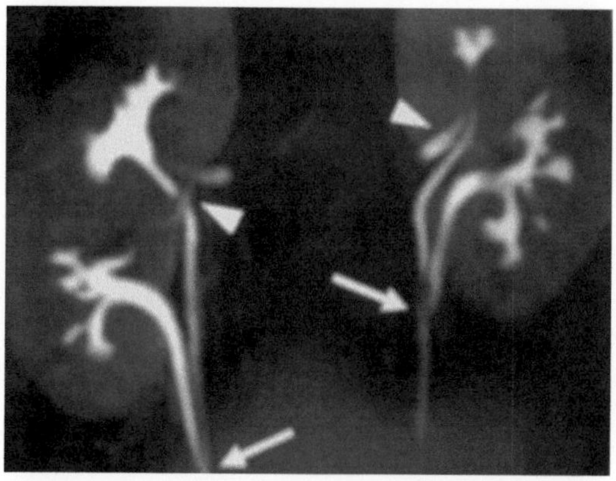

Fig. 1.8 Small diverticula (*triangles*) of upper halves of doubled pelvicalyceal systems of kidneys (*arrows*) in magnetic resonance urograms (Nolte-Erusting et al. [60])

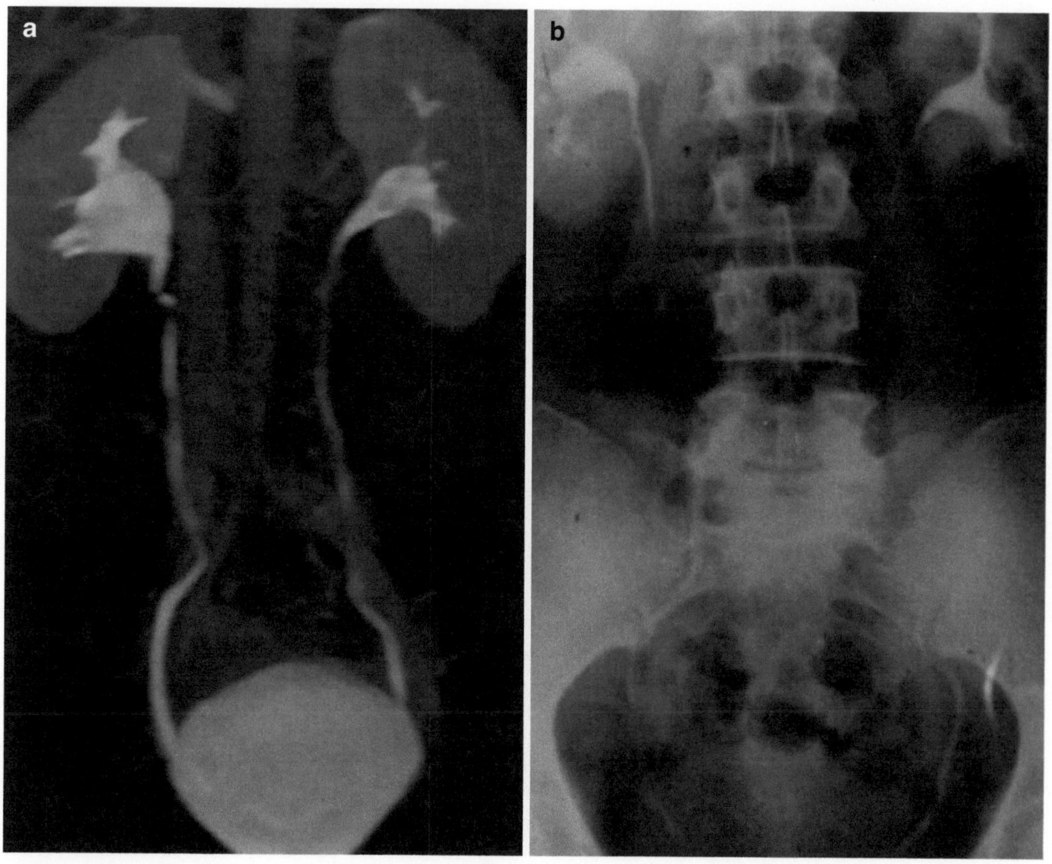

Fig. 1.9 Results of MRU with contrast enhancement (**a**) and of intravenous urography (**b**) done on a 43-year-old kidney donor. Unlike conventional urography, MRU allows to visualize outlines of a normal kidney parenchyma and condition of the upper urinary tract along the whole of its length (El-Diasty et al. [63])

"targeted" USG, will be shifting and has already started to shift to the "first tier" as technical abilities emerge [97].

1.7 Differential Diagnostics

Calyx diverticulum must be differentiated from congenital abnormalities of calyces, namely, tubulomedullar dilatation and medullar hypoplasia or megacalycosis, as well as with isolated hydrocalycosis and tuberculous caverna.

Tubulomedullar dilatation is the expansion of one or more outlet tubules in the renal pyramid. This kind of abnormality can be observed in one, two, and even in all kidney pyramids. Radiographically it appears as a spindle-shaped expansion located in a renal papilla or sometimes a thin duct between the spin-shaped expansion and the calyx opening at the top of the pyramid. This kind of X-ray visual structure can be easily mistaken for papilla necrosis. However, Yu. A. Pytel and I. I. Zolotaryov (1974, 1987) emphasize that in the case of tubulomedullar dilatation, the papilla and fornix stay unchanged. Moreover, image of the expanded tubule as contrasted urine accumulates in it emerges only in an excretory urogram [26, 64].

Medullar hypoplasia (megacalycosis) is an embryonic defect of medullary substance which appears in calyx expansion due to underdevelopment of the final kidney. In case of megacalycosis, pyramids lose their usual shape. Vacant space is left which is overtaken by the minor calyx separated from the cortex only with a thin layer of the underdeveloped pyramid. In excretory urograms, contrast media appears both in the kidney with megacalycosis and in the contralateral kidney at the same time. An abundance of enlarged calyces of triangle or faceted shape is detected which are located in the thickness of kidney parenchyma with their top toward the pelvis. Capacity of expanded calyces exceeds that of pelvis and they are filled slowly. The pelvis is not expanded. Urine drainage is not hindered. Urodynamics of the upper urinary tract is undisturbed. The main difference between calyx diverticulum and megacalycosis lies in its development—it usually appears in one calyx and is much less common in two calyces, unlike megacalycosis which affects all calyces. When it comes to differential diagnostics of calyx diverticula, which are generally found in one or, in very rare cases, in two calyces, and megacalycosis, the latter abnormality, as it follows from its name, can be only multiple on one and on both sides [68–70] (Fig. 1.36).

Calyx diverticulum is often mistaken for *isolated hydrocalycosis*, a much more commonly occurring condition resulting from calyx neck blockade and diminution due to various congenital and acquired processes. According to congenital *hydrocalycosis sizes* can have several degrees from the 1st degree, small upper calyx diverticulum; to the 2nd, when calyx diverticulum cavity can occupy up to 2/3 of the kidney volume; and to the 3rd, when calyx diverticulum cavity can occupy the whole kidney (Fig. 1.10).

Many authors emphasize the necessity to ensure differential diagnostics of *isolated hydrocalycosis* and calyx diverticulum [66, 67]. Ultrasound technique has a low practical efficiency in differential diagnostics of isolated hydrocalycosis and calyx diverticulum. At the same time a series of multiple-view spot excretory urograms as well as cineradiographic visualization allow to clearly observe the stable triangle shape of dilated calyx differentiating it from calyx diverticulum which has a rounded shape. Also a short oblique filling defect is discovered caused by compression from an accessory vessel varying in intensity which changes in width depending on the pelvicalyceal system filling, accessory vessel engorgement, and intra-abdominal pressure (Fig. 1.33).

We did not discover functional lability of diverticulum walls by investigation of urodynamics of pelvicalyceal system and of calyx diverticulum area performed by means of cineradiographic visualization [22]. The same result was obtained by [33, 74] as opposed to V. D. Grund and B. N. Voskresensky [73]. Filling of diverticulum cavity with contrast media was progressing slowly; it flew in from the pelvicalyceal system at different times depending on the length, diameter, and patency of the connecting duct. Small calyceal diverticula were filled almost simultaneously

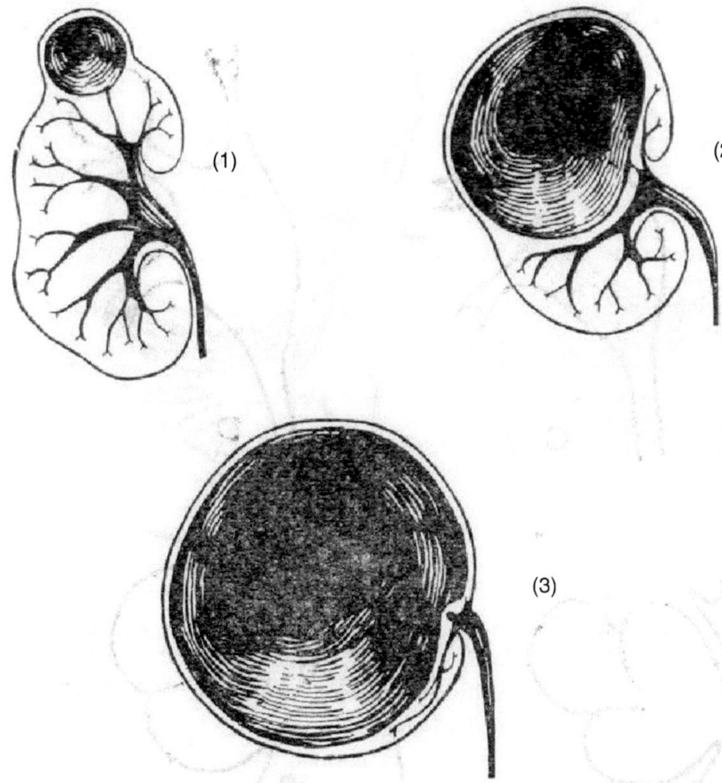

Fig. 1.10 Various degrees of congenital hydrocalycosis; after Pytel and Pugachyov [9])

with the whole pelvicalyceal system; the larger ones got opacified later and were better distinguished in delayed urograms.

Absence of motor activity in calyx diverticulum walls may be explained by the presence of a fibrous capsule around the diverticulum [74] as well as by its location in the depth of the kidney which is a parenchymal organ, unlike alimentary tract diverticula as alimentary tract consists of hollow organs with walls capable of motor activity. This may also explain the absence of enlargement of calyx diverticulum as opposed to hydrocalycosis during a pharmacosonographic test with diuretics.

If contractions are observed during differential diagnostics of calyx diverticulum and isolated hydrocalycosis, this observation confirms the latter. Moreover, ectatic calyx does not have a strictly round shape, and in multiple-view scans, it almost always preserves a triangle shape (Fig. 1.34).

In case of congenital isolated hydrocalycosis, the triangle shape of the calyx is also maintained and usually an abnormal structure of the whole pelvicalyceal system is observed (Figs. 1.35, 1.36, and 1.37). On the contrary, in case of calyx diverticulum, pelvicalyceal system structure is normal.

Radiographic features of calyx diverticulum and of calyx hydrocalycosis are summarized in Table 1.1.

In accordance with data by A. L. Shabad [71], the rate of misidentifying of congenital abnormalities and *tuberculous kidney lesion* in the preadmission stage is 74 %. Seventy one percent of patients with kidney structure abnormalities were erroneously diagnosed with destructive tuberculosis. Pelvicalyceal diverticula in 29.6 % of cases and sponge kidneys in 5.6 % of cases were misidentified with a tuberculous cavern.

"Most often clinicians and radiologists have to differentiate tuberculous cavern with abnormalities of the medullar substance development

Table 1.1 Radiographic features of calyx diverticulum and of calyx hydrocalycosis

Calyx diverticulum	Calyx hydrocalycosis
Most often a rounded single cavity located to the distal side of the fornix usually of an upper calyx with smooth sharp outlines	The shape of the cavity repeating the initial triangle shape of the calyx persists for a long time as far as the most intensive stages
If multiple stones are present, they are grouped in the same way as multiple polished roentgenocontrast stones inside the gall bladder	Generally solitary and repeating the shape of the calyx
A short duct connecting calyx or pelvis with diverticulum which is not always visible	Generally persisting calyx neck demonstrating peristaltic activity
Absence of functional lability of diverticulum walls in cineradiographic images	Cineradiographic visualization reveals contractions of walls of dilated calyx

(megacalyx, megacalycosis, calyx diverticulum, etc.). The greatest similarity of urographic view is between calyx diverticulum and monocavernous tuberculosis (Fig. 1.40). This abnormality is known to be marked by preservation of vestiges of Bellini ducts and presence of Malpighian pyramid located in the cortex. The respective calyx is shaped similar to megacalyx and is connected with the neck of the major calyx or with the pelvis by means of a narrow passage. Localization of the calyx and the structure of its connection with the urinary tract can be determined by multiaxis radiography. Localization of solitary caverns is performed in a similar way. It is commonly known that a long existing cavern has smooth walls and outlines and may contain secondary concrements. It should be noted that in case of excretory urography the cavern is filled in the retrograde way (selective pyelography phenomenon described by Olsson [76]), it means while the pelvicalyceal system is sharply contrast the cavern cavity is filled in the retrograde way, as seen from delayed images, since cicatrical walls of the cavern do not egest the contrast medium. In case of medullary substance abnormalities a distinct and timely cavity opacification is observed since the abnormal area is functionally sound. Is a concrement is present in the calyx diverticulum its differentiation from a calcified tuberculosis focus is very difficult."

Table 1.2 Radiographic features of calyx diverticulum and destructive renal tuberculosis (Grund and Voskresensky [73])

Calyx diverticulum	Destructive tuberculosis
Usually a solitary cavity with smooth walls is present	More often multilocular focus with irregular walls
Presence of solitary, multiple in less frequent cases, *polished* radiopaque stones inside the diverticulum	Often tyroid mass is detected
A short duct connecting the calyx or pelvis and diverticulum	Calyx neck is tapered; the calyx can be misshapen or ablated
Preservation of motor activity in the marginal area and in the diverticulum area which is observed at cineradiographic visualization	Dysmotility, more often of the cavity itself, then in the marginal area, as observed at cineradiographic visualization
Absence of radiographic dynamics after the test therapy	Upon application of specific therapy, radiographic dynamics is observed in the form of exclusion or calcification of the tuberculous focus

Based on 11 patients (four patients with sponge kidney, seven with megapolycalycosis), apart from overdiagnosis of kidney tuberculosis in one patient, bilateral megapolycalycosis complicated with the left kidney tuberculous papillitis was discovered (the first description in the world literature!) (V. S. Gagarinov, I. S. Kamyshan, and V. M. Pogrebinsky) [75]. In this case only a complex analysis of radiographic and bacteriological data and of provocative tuberculin tests helped to determine the correct diagnosis.

Although our experience and available literature contain no descriptions of calyx diverticulum combined with kidney tuberculosis, the abovementioned observation confirms a possibility of such combination!

Some authors emphasize that "calyx diverticulum or tuberculous cavern can be diagnosed correctly only by exception" [70] (Figs. 1.38, 1.39, 1.40, and 1.41). Radiographic features of calyx diverticulum and destructive renal tuberculosis are summarized in Table 1.2 [73].

In rare cases as noted by Fr. Brunzema [24], calyx diverticulum in urographic presentation must be differentiated from *disintegrating renal tumor which has broken into the pelvicalyceal system.*

This situation can result from a traumatic or, which is very rare, spontaneous rupture that can happen not only to a tumor but also to a simple kidney cyst, when, apart from hematoma formation, its rupture takes place with release into the pelvicalyceal system [37, 80]. In this case against retrograde filling of the formed cavity with a contrast agent, excretory urogram may display a presentation similar to calyx diverticulum while ultrasound and CAT data may simulate renal tumor picture.

A patient with a traumatic rupture of a simple renal cyst accompanied by release into the pelvicalyceal system which looked like calyx diverticulum in an excretory urogram and simulated tumorlike picture in sonograms and CAT images is described below (Fig. 1.44).

A 73-year-old woman fell on her left side and got pains in the left portion of her lumbar region in combination with multiple painless gross hematuria. During a primary USG examination in a polyclinic, a rounded formation was discovered in the upper segment of the left kidney with a diameter about 5.0 cm and nonhomogenous echostructure which was interpreted as a tumor. In accordance with CAT results, the formation had a nonhomogenous structure with an obscurely visible sac and displayed a low ability of contrast agent accumulation. The conclusion is as follows: Tumor must be differentiated with hemorrhage and a traumatic renal hematoma. EU, performed after USG and CAT, displayed an intensive retrograde opacification of the cavity in the upper segment of the left kidney, diameter about 5 cm, with increase seen in delayed images, which was not typical for tumor but was similar to the cavity of a large diverticulum of an upper calyx. During a thorough repeated history taking, it was discovered that 12 years ago during a preclinical abdominal USG, a large cyst was discovered in the upper segment of the left kidney of the patient. At the same time, EU was done that revealed indirect indicators of an expansive process in the upper segment of the left kidney which was pushing pelvicalyceal system down to the bottom. A retrospective analysis of provided archive sonograms and excretory urograms as compared to the new data, namely, urographic presentation of a retrograde opacification of the cavity connected with the pelvicalyceal system, gave grounds for suggesting a traumatic rupture of a kidney cyst with its release into the pelvicalyceal system. The diagnosis became evident upon a retrospective analysis of archive ultrasound and urographic data which confirmed a renal cyst in the anamnesis as well as upon shrinkage of the ambiguous renal formation from 5.0 to 1.5 cm in control sonograms in 2 months after the trauma.

We would like to draw attention to the fact that calyx diverticulum is often diagnosed by means of exclusion of the abovementioned diseases and in this process both retrospective analysis of available data and, in ambiguous cases, dynamic observation are of importance.

1.8 Treatment

Treatment depends on respective size and localization of calyx diverticulum, functional state of the kidney, and pyelonephritis and lithogenesis which complicate this abnormality. For patients who have no health complaints, no treatment is required; however they must be under dynamic observation.

In case of pains and frequent pyelonephritis recrudescence, various kinds of surgical aid are recommended: (1) calyceal cyst resection with celiorrhaphy, (2) discission and draining of the calyx diverticulum cavity with celiorrhaphy, and (3) partial nephrectomy which is justified in those cases when the cyst is located in the upper or lower kidney segment and is a focus of lithogenesis and source of infection. Partial nephrectomy should include resection of the focus of the calyceal neck obstruction. Pyelolithotomy in case of calyx diverticulum undiagnosed prior to surgery may result in failure to remove the stone from the diverticulum by means of conventional surgery due to technical limitations (Fig. 1.26).

For the recent decades, a lot of reports have been made about application of endoscopic surgery, percutaneous nephrolithomy (PCNL), and remote or contact lithotripsy of concrements in calyx diverticulum cavity [81–91].

Kikuchi E., Sumitomo M., and Hatakeyama N. et al. [92] stated that before numerous reports described conventional surgical methods for treatment of calyx diverticula with calcium milk, but later those aggressive methods were replaced

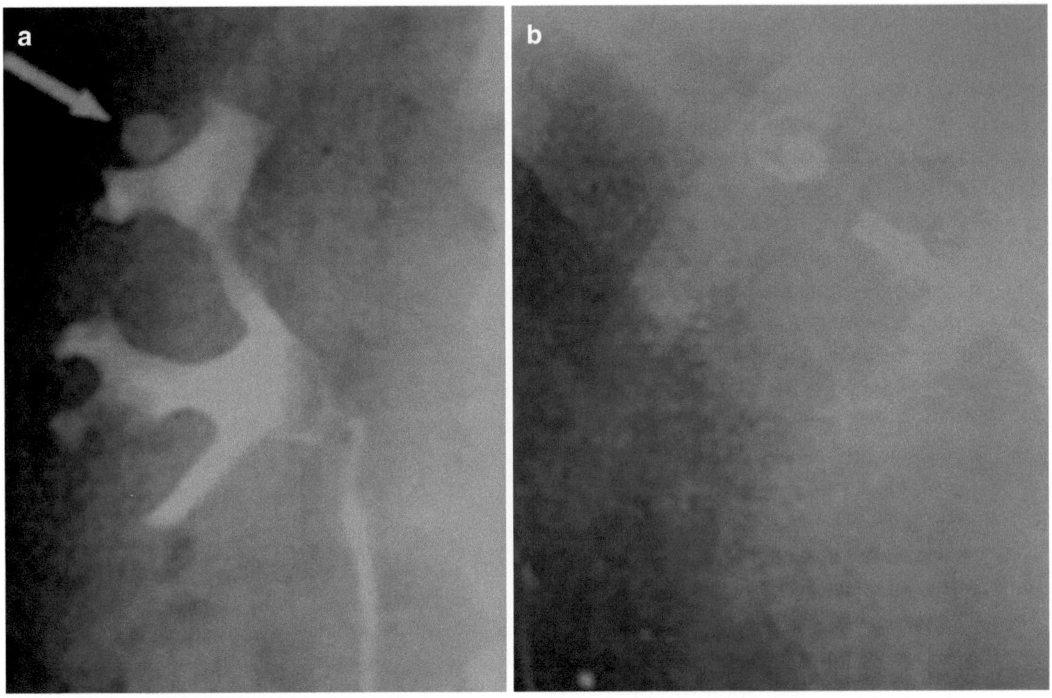

Fig. 1.11 (**a**, **b**) A stone in a small diverticulum in an upper calyx of the right kidney, removed by means of endoscopic dilatation of the neck and contact lithotripsy with a holmium laser (After Andersson [91])

by percutaneous methods and thus a patient was reported with rupture of calyx diverticulum containing small renal stones and calcium milk that were successfully removed by means of endourologic procedures (Fig. 1.11a, b).

As it was mentioned before, stones can be removed from calyx diverticulum by means of remote or contact lithotripsy and percutaneous nephrolithomy (PCNL) (if possible) or by means of retrograde urethroscopy. An additional method for diverticular stone removal is videoendoscopic retroperitoneal surgery [36]. In case of limited communication between the diverticulum and renal urinoexcretory system, crushed stones will stay in their initial position. In such patients, symptoms may disappear after the first stone crushing [91].

Nephrectomy is justified in rare cases, only if a malignant growth, diffuse purulent pyelonephritis, or tuberculosis develops in the cyst.

Professor Arthur Smith, president of the World Endourological Society, USA, in his report Treatment of Calyx Diverticula at the 1st Russian Congress of Endourology (Moscow, 2008) gave the following definition of calyx diverticulum—it is a nonsecretory isolated intrarenal calyx connected with the pelvicalyceal system by a narrow neck which does not contain collecting tubules and papillae and is filled with urine passively from contiguous sections of renal collection system. Diverticulum size varies from 0.5 to 7.5 cm, and size above 2 cm is considered large; calyx diverticulum can be located in any segment of the kidney. Professor Smith divides calyx diverticula in the following groups in accordance with their etiology: congenital, diverticula which appear on the 5–8th week of gestation due to uncompleted regression process of ureteral tubules of the 3–4th order, and acquired, by means of a blunt kidney trauma, acquired obstruction of calyx infundibula, and dyssynergia of sphincters around minor calyces (in theory).

Calyx Diverticulum Classification: *This includes* type I diverticula connected with minor calyces or infundibula and type II diverticula starting from the pelvis or major calyces; generally they have a more prominent clinical presentation and are located in the middle segment of the kidney.

Clinical Presentation: Mostly asymptomatic, discovered casually, in 1/3 of cases, diverticula are clinically displayed as pains, hematuria, urinary tract infections, and urine stasis which causes diverticulum dilatation, and as a result, crystallization of calcium salts may develop, both without and with lithogenesis (calcium stones), concomitant infection may arise, and passage of stones through a narrow duct into the calyx causes pain and hematuria. Lithogenesis in calyx diverticulum cavity is detected in 10–40 % of calyceal diverticulum cases. The size of stones ranges from microscopic calcium suspension or mass of small concrements to several large stones; *calcium suspension is a colloidal solution of calcium salts (carbonates, phosphates, and oxalates) and can be both radionegative and radiopositive.*

Indications for treatment are as follows: persistent pains, recurrent urinary tract infections, recurrent lithogenesis, hematuria, progressing kidney destruction, and calyceal diverticulum size over 2.5 cm. The following treatment principles must be followed: attempt must be made to remove the concrement, provide the cavity obliteration and expansion of the diverticular infundibulum. RL may mitigate symptoms, but this will not eliminate the diverticulum and does not guarantee improvement of drainage from its cavity; this may provoke recurrence of lithogenesis. The most effective methods are percutaneous ones; in case of small size of calyceal diverticulum, ureteroscopy is used, and in case of large diverticula which protrude to the anterior renal surface, laparoscopy is applied. *But the real key to success emphasized by A. Smith is the individual approach to every patient.*

In summary, detection of such symptoms as *calcium milk*, *rattlebag syndrome*, and *twinking artifact* by means of ultrasound and X-ray imaging helps to fulfill diagnostics and choose treatment strategy in case concrements or calcium milk is present in the calyx diverticulum cavity, namely, observation, remote lithotripsy, or surgery [93].

1.9 Author's Data and Clinical Examples

In 1989–2010 we observed 52 cases of calyx diverticulum in 51 patients. Fifty patients had solitary diverticula. Thirty two patients had calyx diverticulum in the right kidney and 20 patients had calyx diverticulum in the left kidney including one patient with two calyceal diverticula in the duplex left kidney (Fig. 1.19). In 37 patients calyx diverticulum was located in upper calyx, in five patients in middle calyx, and in seven patients in lower calyx, and two patients had pelvis diverticulum (Figs. 1.16 and 1.17).

In the great majority of patients, diverticula were discovered "accidentally" during EU or USG tests. It should be mentioned that an ultrasound diagnosis of calyx diverticulum or USG-based suggestions about the presence of calyx diverticulum prior to EU were made only by doctors who had previous experience of calyx diverticulum diagnostics. The majority of patients during primary USG examination were diagnosed with pyelo-, calycectasis and caliectasis with or without concrements or "cysts with or without suspension."

Thirty patients were subject to dynamic ultrasound observation, one female patient had a RL of a small concrement, and nine patients got conservative treatment of detected concomitant inflammatory diseases of the kidneys and upper urinary tract.

Out of seven patients with calcium milk phenomenon observed by us, only three patients got a correct diagnosis upon USG examination. Other patients were offered or given ineffective RL treatment for "calyx stones."

The biggest number of patients [5] with calcium milk in the calyx diverticulum cavity was observed by us during the last 3 years when RL rooms started operating in our clinics. All patients were directed to the clinic for RL of "calyceal concrements." In all patients, calyx diverticula were "accidental" USG findings which were interpreted like pyelocaliectasis and caliectasis with concrements. Upon analyzing the provided sonogram and urogram and performing repeated multiple-view spot USG with an obligatory scanning in the vertical position, we had no grounds to question the diagnosed calyx diverticulum with calcium milk; thus there was no need to perform or repeat excretory urography. The so-called twinking artifact at USDG was detected in three patients with calcium milk in calyx diverticulum cavity (Fig. 1.26).

Among five patients observed by us, one patient was recommended to have a RL in one of Moscow urological clinics based only on renal USG which was interpreted as a concrement in a dilated calyx (Fig. 1.17). Four patients appointed for "RL of renal concrements" were diagnosed with calcium milk in the calyx diverticulum which allowed to dispense with the planned RL.

Five patients were diagnosed with stones in the calyx diverticulum. One patient got a confirmed diagnosis of minor concrement in the calyx diverticulum cavity and rattlebox symptom only after multiple-view USG and CAT examinations. Prior to that during preclinical abdominal USG, the results were interpreted as calyx stones, while no stones were visible in the overall radiogram of urinary system and in the excretory urogram (Fig. 1.20). One female patient had a RL of a stone in the calyx diverticulum with incomplete removal of concrement fragments within 2 weeks; the patient is still under observation. Other four patients with stones in the calyx diverticulum due to their asymptomatic presence undergo ultrasound monitoring once a year.

We observed a female patient with a stone in the calyx diverticulum who got a wrong interpretation of USG and EU data obtained in a nonspecialized clinic which concluded that it was a stone in a constricted upper calyx. Only thanks to SCTU, an unaltered upper calyx was detected with clarifications of its calyx diverticulum neck anatomy, namely, its diminution and arch bending with the arch top pointing upward (Fig. 1.24). This allowed to dispense with initially appointed RL and recommend further observation or contact lithotripsy with a preliminary endoscopic discission of the diverticulum neck.

During recent years in connection with common application of various renal ultrasound examination techniques (USG), "accidental" calyx diverticulum detection has become more frequent (Figs. 1.12, 1.13, 1.14, and 1.15). At primary USG, these findings are usually interpreted as isolated hydrocalycosis. If lithogenesis or calcium milk in the calyx diverticulum is present, they are mistaken for stones in calyces. Correct diagnostics of calcium milk is very important in view of the fact that unlike concrements it does not require lithotripsy and is not sensitive to that. We observed a female patient who was suggested to have a RL for a "large concrement in an ectatic calyx" based on USG and EU data, and only a multiple-view SCT and an upright radiography helped to detect a clear horizontal level created by calcium milk in a large calyx diverticulum (Fig. 1.30).

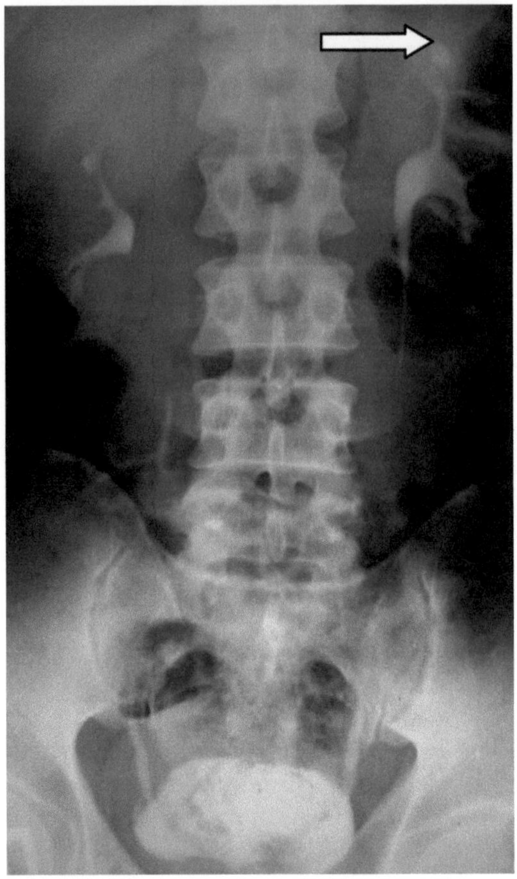

Fig. 1.12 An "accidental" detection of a small diverticulum (*arrow*) in an upper calyx of the left kidney (not discovered by USG) in an excretory urogram in the 10th min; the test was carried out for the urinary bladder trauma (band-like defects present in it due to blood clots)

We must emphasize that it is very important not to limit diagnostics of calyx diverticulum with calcium milk and lithogenesis to USG as X-ray technique is also mandatory. The following radiological methods can be used: spot radiology on a patient in the horizontal and vertical position, EU with cineradiographic monitoring, and (or) multiple-view SCT/MSCT and SCTU/

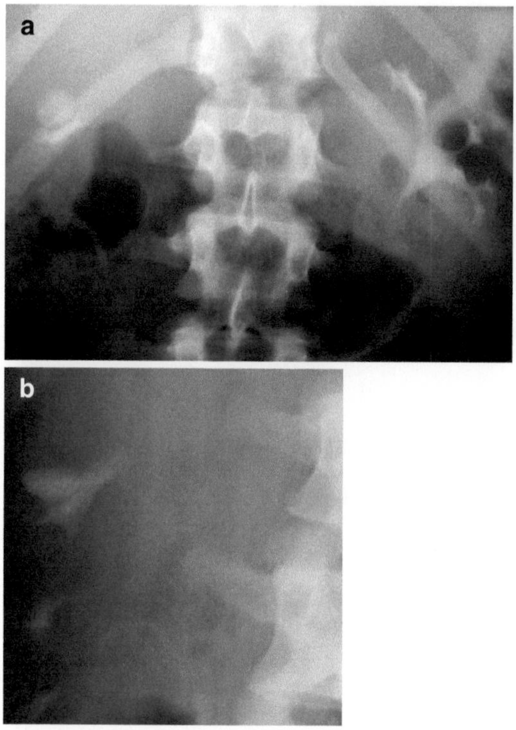

Fig. 1.13 (a, b) A typical diverticulum in the right kidney upper calyx in an excretory urogram, 10th min, and in a spot excretory urogram, 11th min, on the right, with the patient in vertical position

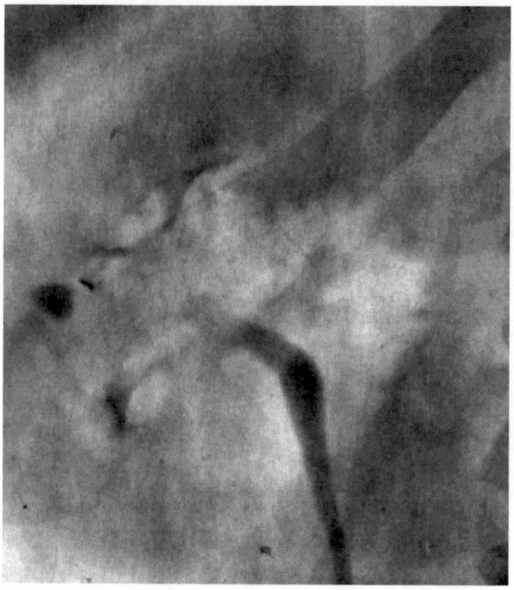

Fig. 1.14 A fragment of an excretory urogram, 15th min, done under cineradiographic monitoring resulting in a typical "accidental" discovery of a small diverticulum of the right kidney middle calyx

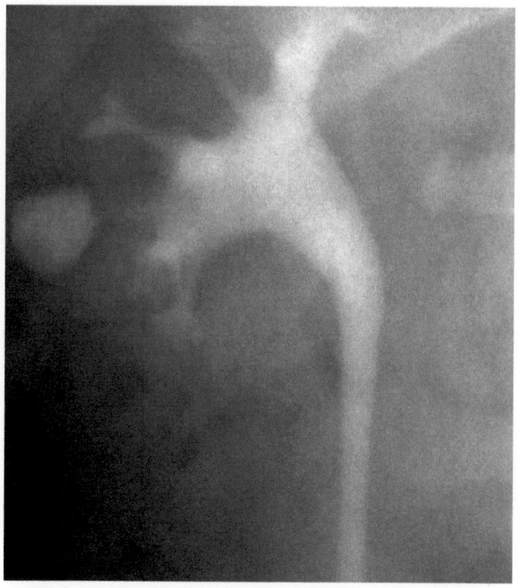

Fig. 1.15 An "accidental discovery" of a typical diverticulum in the right kidney lower calyx in an excretory urogram, 7th min, done for the left side renal colic

MSCTU. By using these methods, necessity of RL as well as possibility of stone fragment removal can be determined or necessity of contact lithotripsy with preceding endoscopic dilatation of the calyx diverticulum neck.

1.10 Clinical Examples: Author's Observations (Figs. 1.12, 1.13, 1.14, 1.15, 1.16, 1.17, 1.18, 1.19, 1.20, 1.21, 1.22, 1.23, 1.24, 1.25, 1.26, 1.27, 1.28, 1.29, 1.30, 1.31, 1.32, 1.33, 1.34, 1.35, 1.36, 1.37, 1.38, 1.39, 1.40, 1.41, 1.42, 1.43, and 1.44)

1.11 Urinary Tract Diverticula Diagnostics and Treatment Algorithms

The algorithm of ultrasound and X-ray diagnostics for a *noncomplicated calyx or pelvis diverticulum is in our opinion as follows*:

- When a typical ultrasound presentation of a renal calyx or pelvis diverticulum is discovered

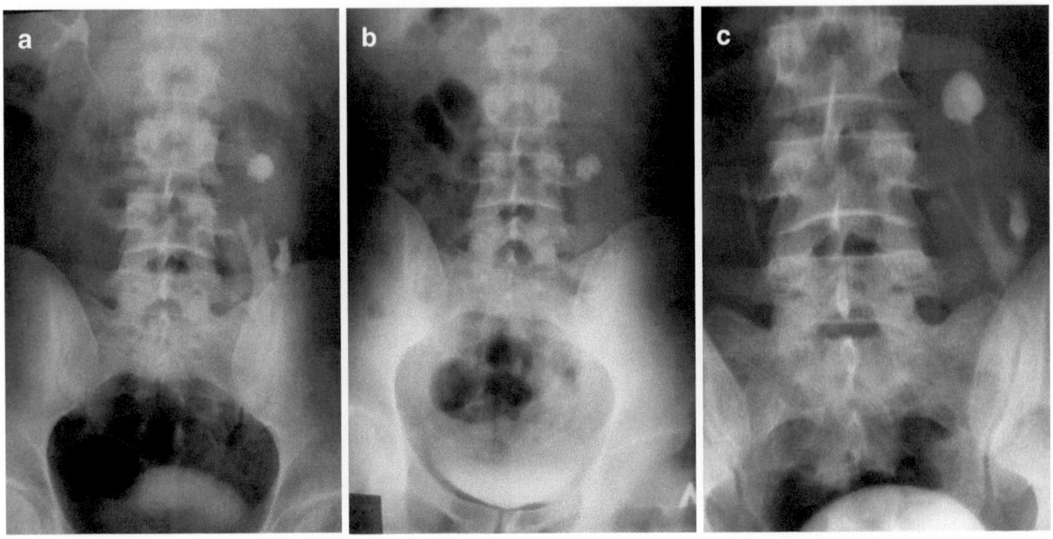

Fig. 1.16 A diverticulum in an upper calyx of the left kidney with lumbar ectopia and uncompleted rotation, an "accidental" finding during examination for lumbar pain in a 26-year-old patient: (**a**) excretory urogram, 10th min; (**b**) upright excretory urogram, 11th min; (**c**) a fragment of excretory urogram, 60th min

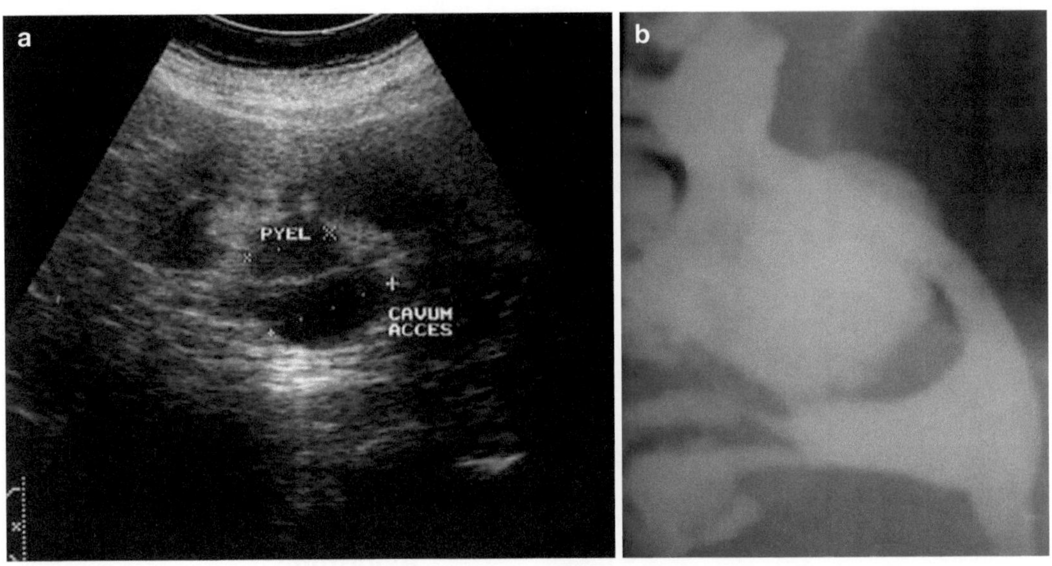

Fig. 1.17 Large diverticulum of the right kidney pelvis, in a sonogram and a retrograde pyelogram: (**a**) a large rounded echo-free cavity located near the pelvis; (**b**) an additional cavity which compresses the pelvis and pushing calyces and the pelvis archwise apart

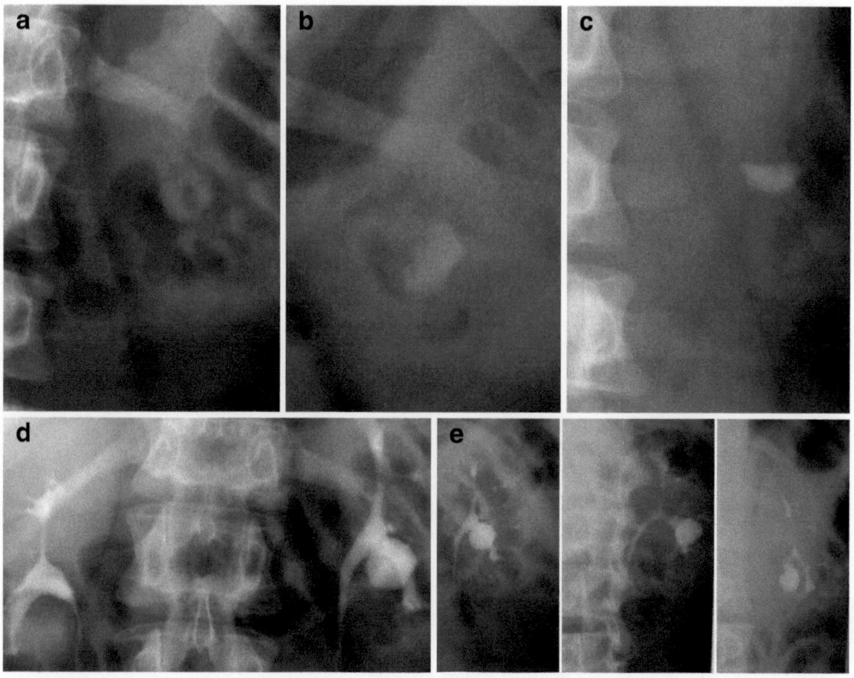

Fig. 1.18 Left kidney diverticulum with calcium milk (several seances of RL was performed for the "stone" in the left kidney in a urological clinic of Saint Petersburg): (**a–c**) spot images of the left kidney taken in the horizontal faceup and facedown position and in the vertical position; (**d**, **e**) excretory urogram, 10th min, and a series of spot multiple-view excretory urograms of the left kidney, 11th min

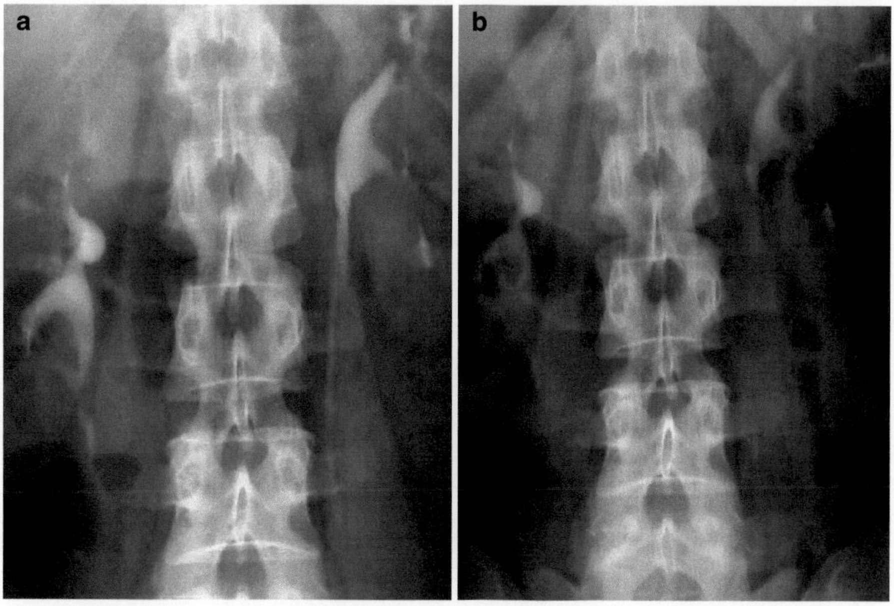

Fig. 1.19 Diverticulum in the right kidney pelvis as displayed in excretory urograms, 10th and 45th min: (**a**) an additional ovoid cavity connected with the upper pelvis segment; (**b**) a more intensive opacification of the pelvis diverticulum cavity in the 45th min

Fig. 1.20 Diverticula (*arrows*) in the upper and lower calyces of the doubled pelvicalyceal system of the left kidney in an excretory urosonogram, 15th min

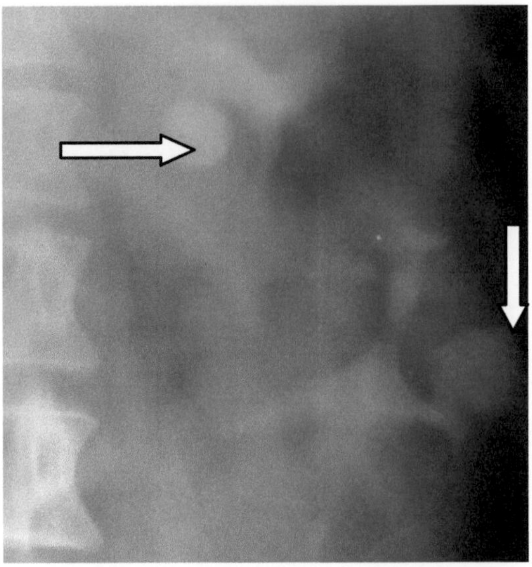

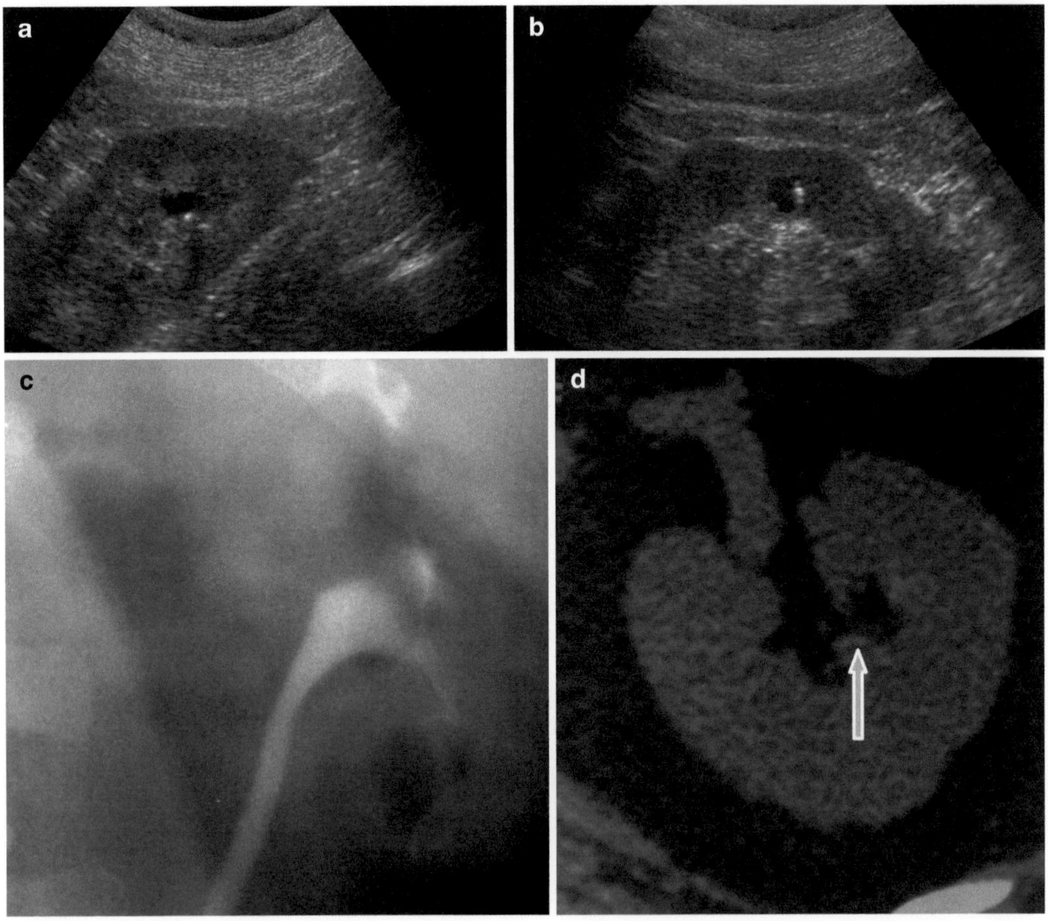

Fig. 1.21 Small stones in the calyx diverticulum as displayed in sonograms, excretory urogram, and plain computer tomogram: (**a**, **b**) shifting of small concrements in the calyx diverticulum cavity when the patient is turning on the right side (rattlebox symptom); (**c**) middle calyx has an anterior orientation, its fornices and concrements not visible; (**d**) several small intensive concrements (*arrow*) in the fornical region of an upper calyx

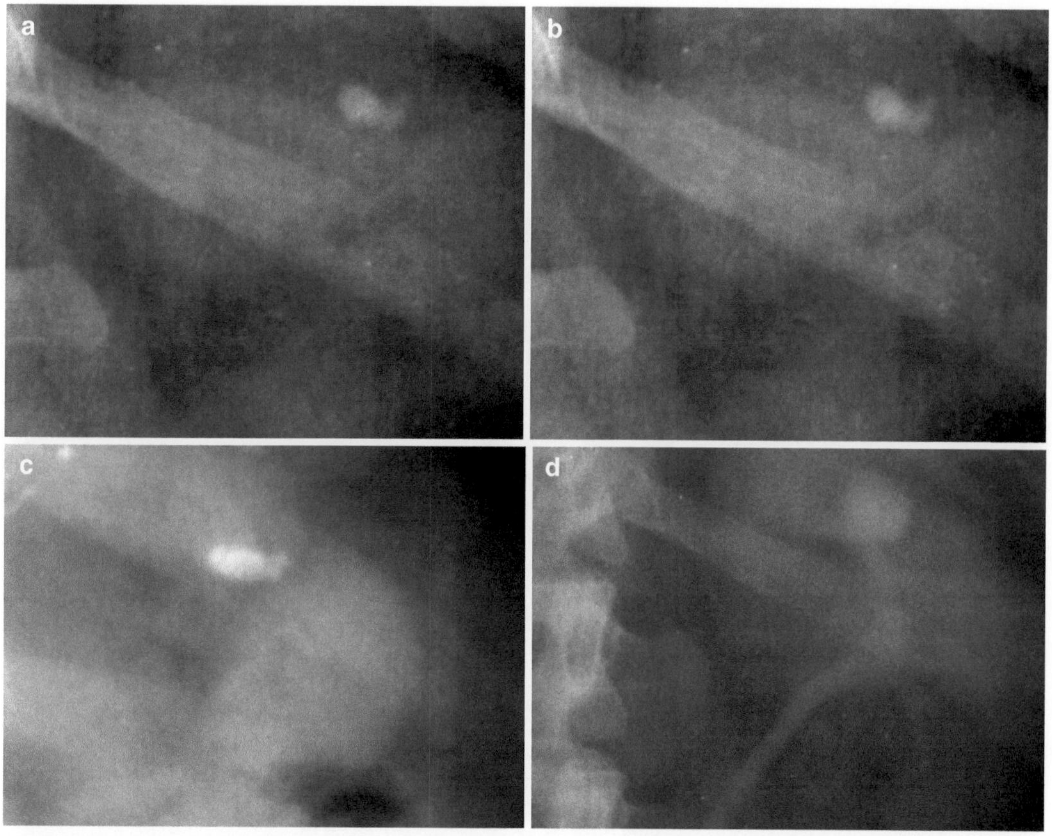

Fig. 1.22 Small stones in diverticulum cavity in an upper calyx of the left kidney: (**a–c**) stone shifting in spot plain images in the horizontal faceup and facedown positions and in the upright position (rattlebox symptom); (**d**) a typical diverticulum presentation in the fragment of an excretory urogram, 25th min

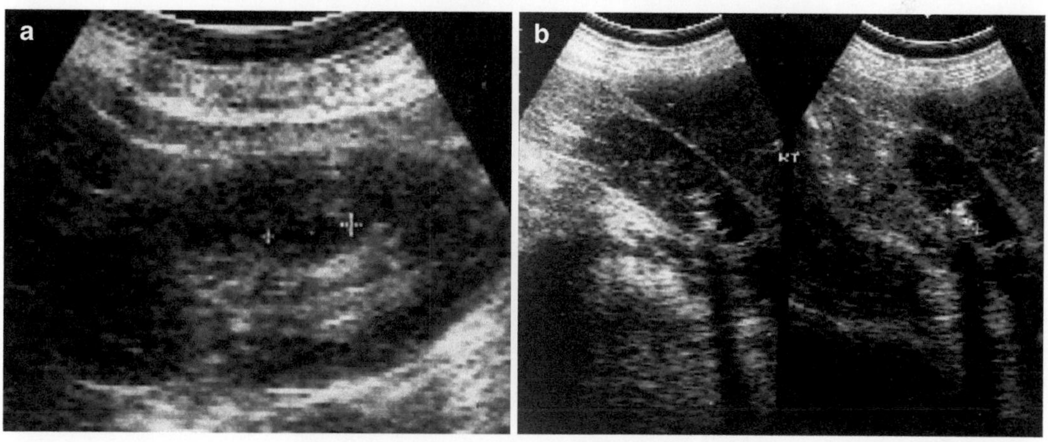

Fig. 1.23 Diverticulum in an upper calyx of the right kidney with concrements: (**a**) echo-producing element with an acoustic shadow in a sonogram taken from patient lying on the right side; (**b**) echo-free element in a sonogram taken from the back; (**c, d**) the same patient, spot overall and excretory urograms

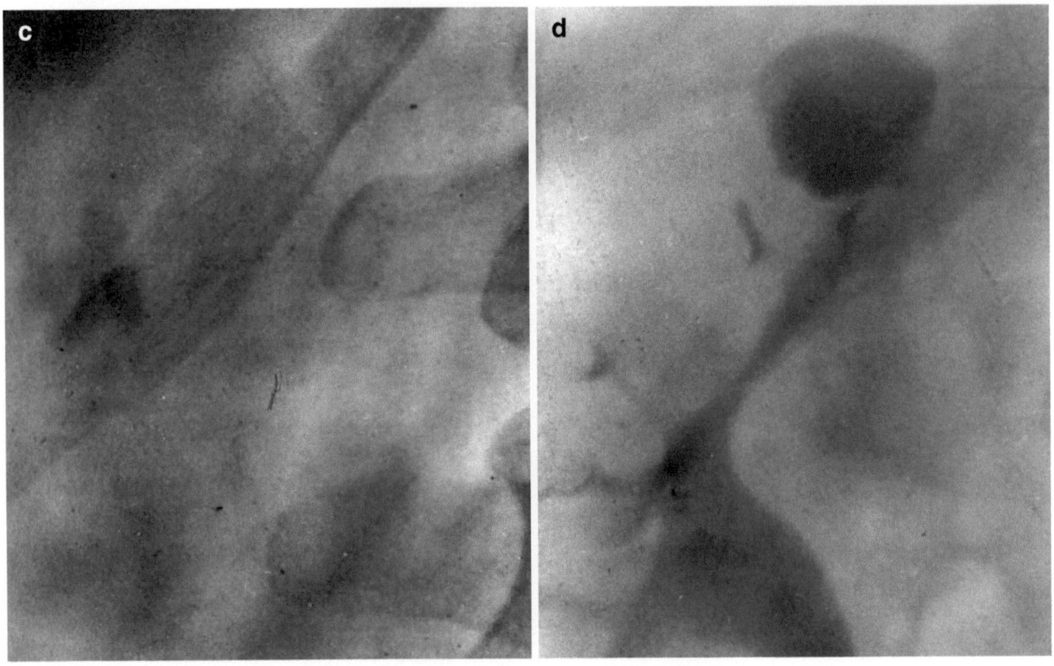

Fig. 1.23 (continued)

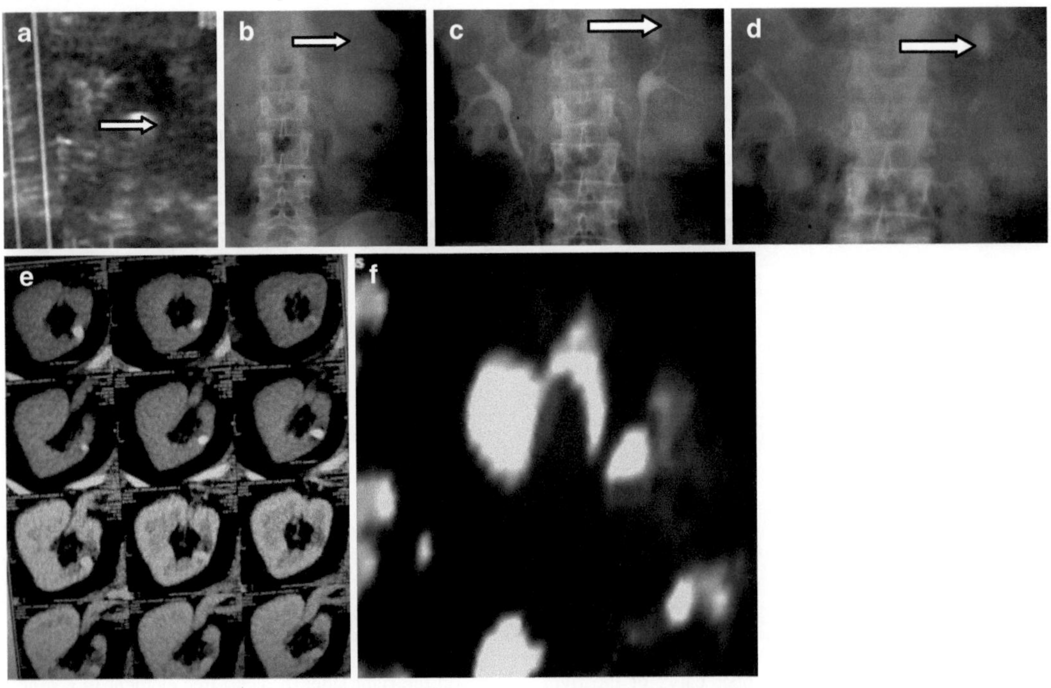

Fig. 1.24 Stone in diverticulum in an upper calyx of the left kidney which was interpreted as a stone (*arrows*) in the upper kidney: (**a**) in a sonogram; (**b**) in an overall radiogram of the urinary system; (**c, d**) excretory urograms of the same female patient, the 10th and 45th min after injection of the contrast agent—opacification of the diverticulum cavity (*arrows*) to the medial side of the unaltered upper calyx; (**d, e**) a series of plain SCT grams and an SCT urogram of the same female patient; (**f**) a stone in the parenchyma of the upper medial segment of the kidney; (**e**) the concrement "disappears" on the background of the contrast medium in the diverticulum cavity

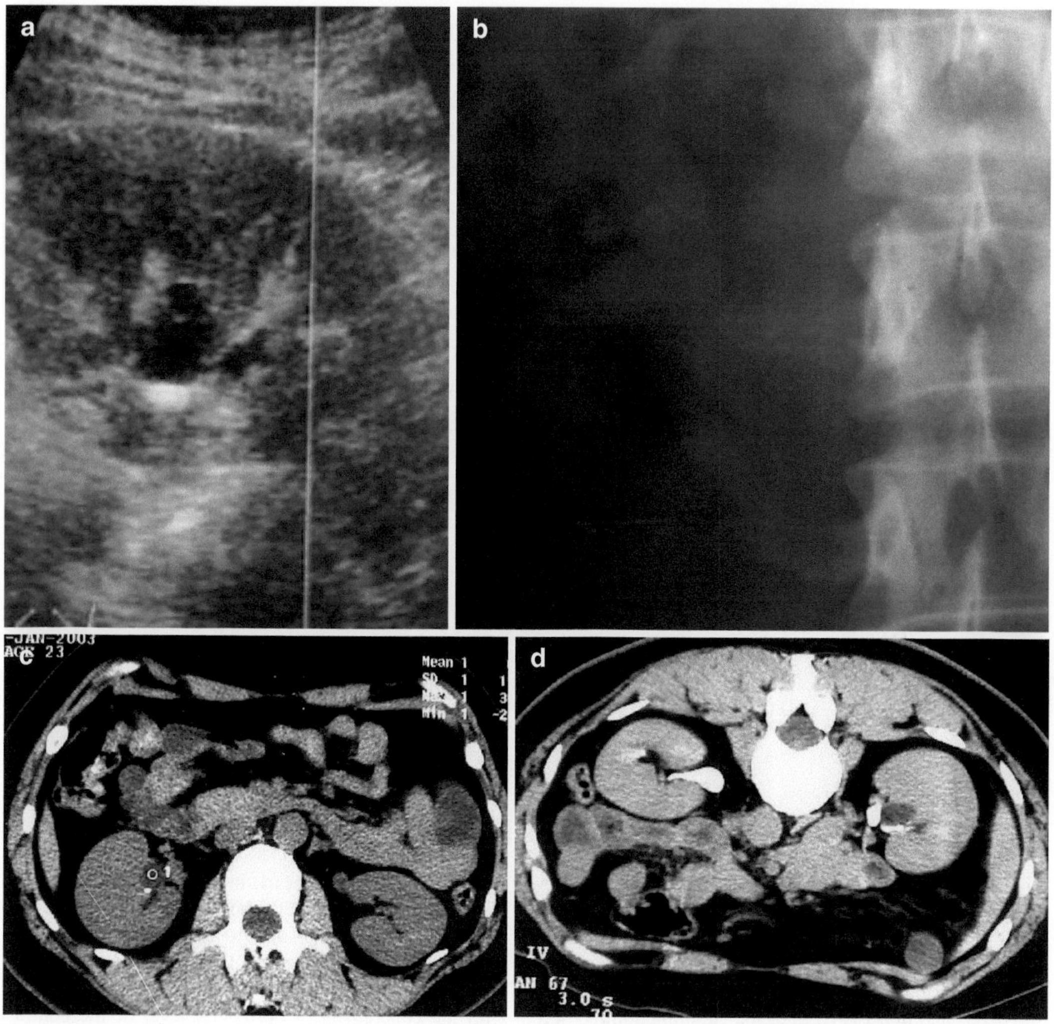

Fig. 1.25 A small stone in diverticulum in a middle calyx of the right kidney and a parapelvic cyst of the left kidney: (**a**) in a sonogram; (**b**) in a spot image; (**c**, **d**) in computer tomograms taken with face up and face down

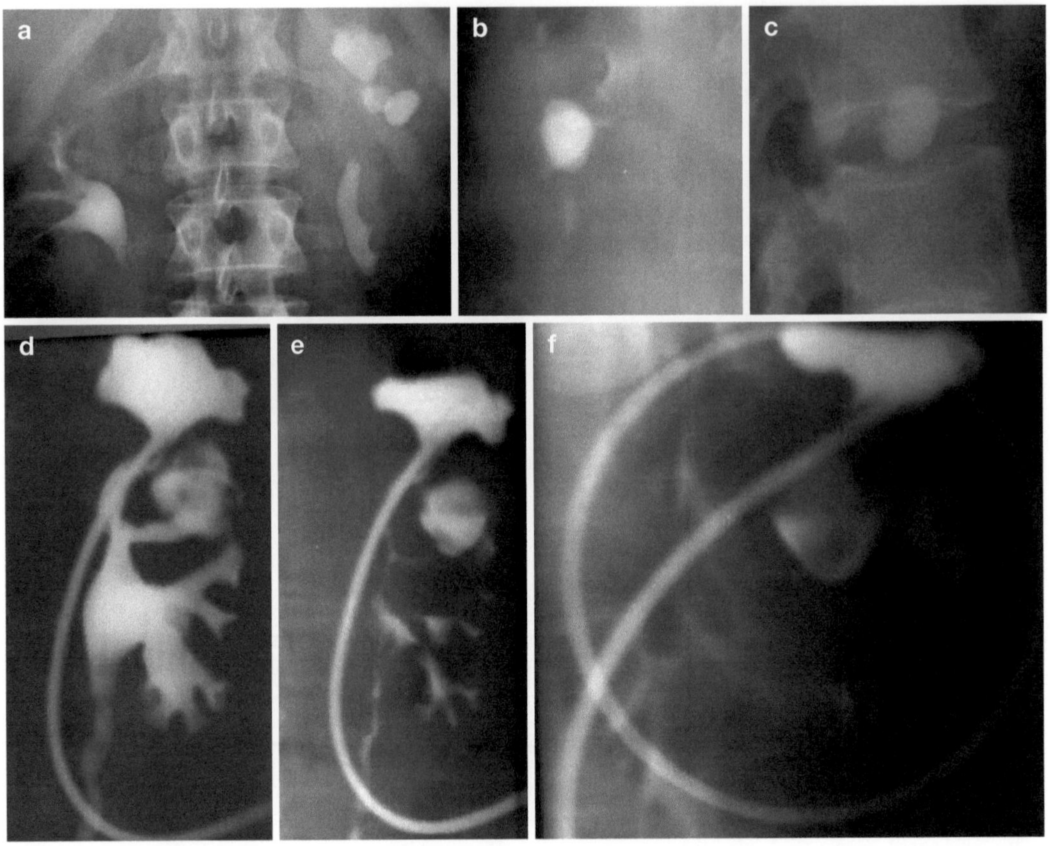

Fig. 1.26 A large stone in the diverticulum in an upper calyx of the left kidney which was failed to remove at pyelolithotomy performed for stones in the pelvis and upper calyces: (**a**) in an excretory urogram, in the 10th min, prior to a surgery, coral calculi are detected in the pelvis and upper calyces of the "nonfunctioning" left kidney; (**b**, **c**) in spot images made in the frontal and side projection of the left kidney after surgery, a remaining concrement can be seen; (**d**) in the antegrade pyelogram taken from the patient in the horizontal position, the concrement is located in an additional rounded cavity of the upper calyx diverticulum; (**e**, **f**) in the antegrade pyelogram taken from the patient in the vertical position along with the concrement, a horizontal level of the contrast agent can be seen in the cavity of the upper calyx diverticulum

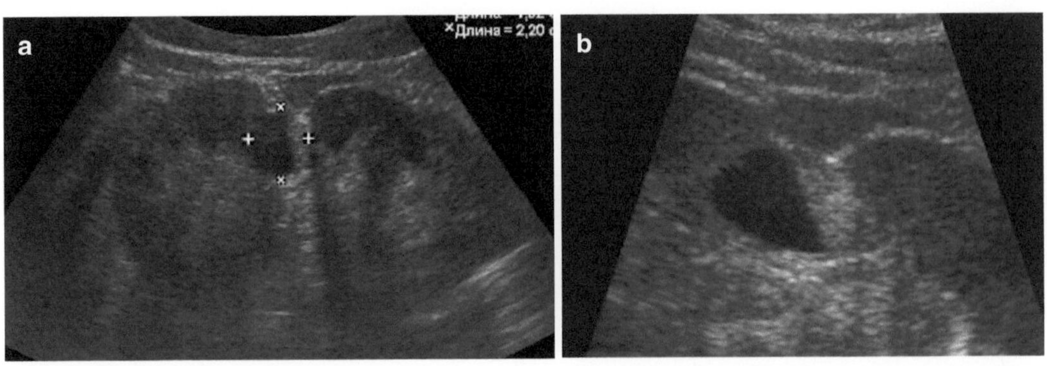

Fig. 1.27 Multiple-view sonograms taken from a patient lying with face up and on the right side and USDG of the left kidney of the patient with calcium milk in the cavity of diverticulum in an upper calyx of the left kidney: (**a**–**c**) a moving boundary between the echo-producing and echo-free components in the diverticulum cavity; (**d**) twinking artifact detected during color Doppler mapping

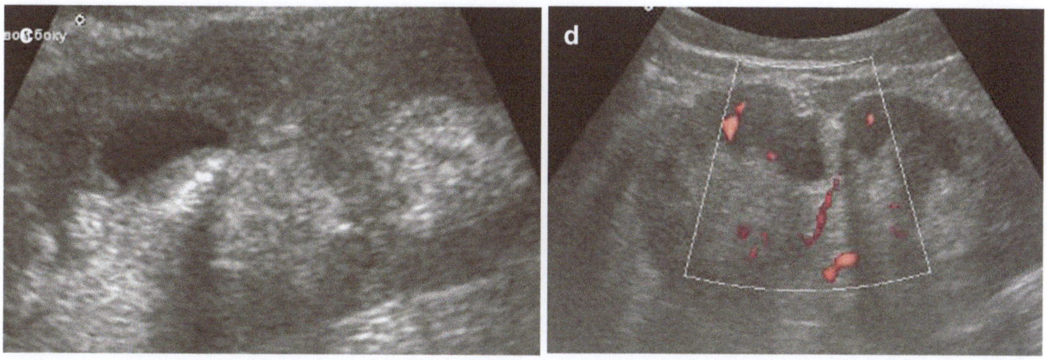

Fig. 1.27 (continued)

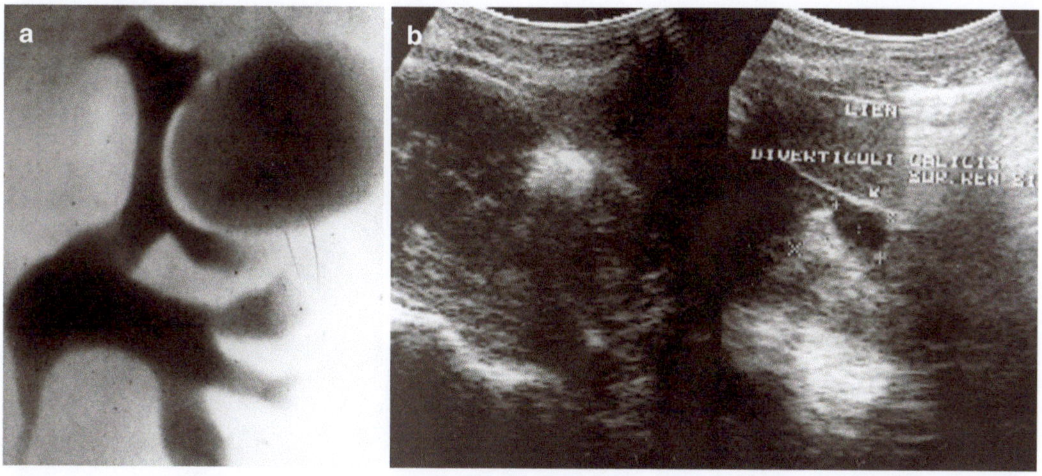

Fig. 1.28 (**a**) Large diverticulum in an upper calyx of the right kidney in an excretory urogram and, (**b**) calcium milk phenomenon in the cavity of the same diverticulum in sonograms taken from patient lying on the right side

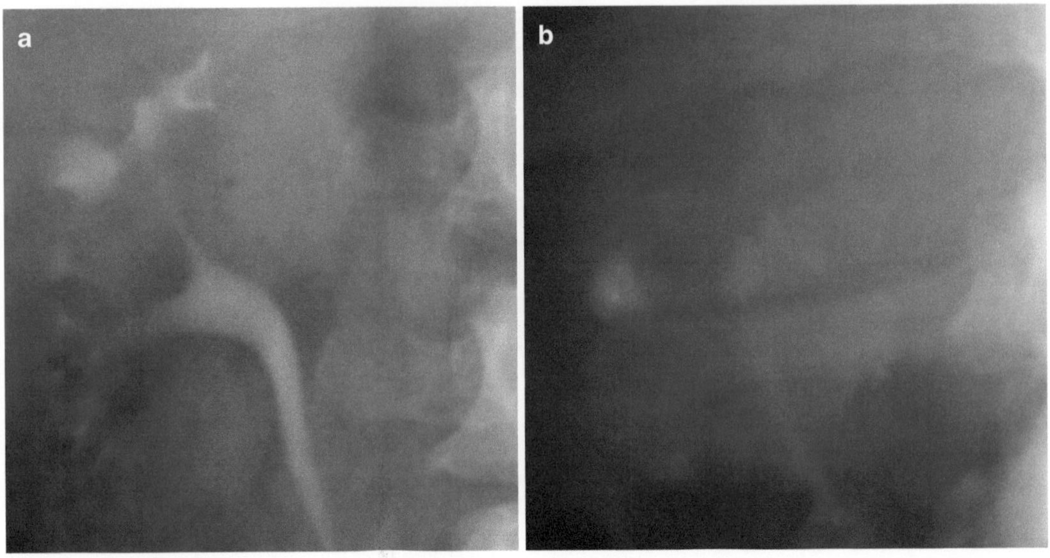

Fig. 1.29 Diverticulum in an upper calyx of the right kidney in excretory urograms: (**a**) horizontal level in the calyx diverticulum cavity is not detected in the 10th min (faceup); (**b**) in the 45th min (with a slight turning on the right side), a meniscus-like right outline is detected due to the presence of calcium milk in the calyx diverticulum cavity

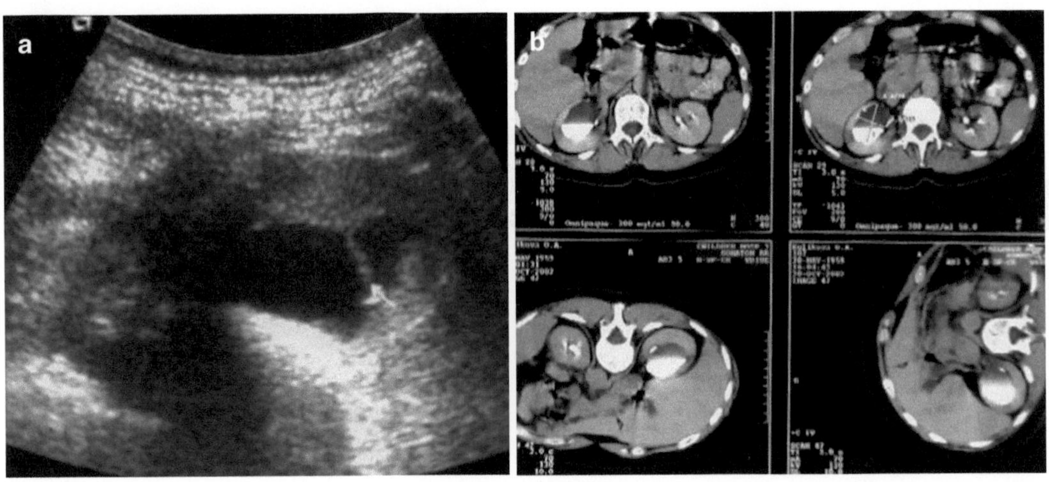

Fig. 1.30 A giant diverticulum in an upper calyx of the right kidney (in accordance with primary USG, a "stone" in the pelvis was diagnosed and RL was recommended). (**a**) Multiple-view USG in a urological clinic—a giant diverticulum in an upper calyx of the right kidney with calcium milk in it which creates a shifting horizontal level between the echo-free and the echo-producing contents of the diverticulum cavity. (**b**) A series of multiple-view CAT grams from the same female patient with face up, face down, and on the right side—a horizontal shifting level in the diverticulum cavity due to calcium milk in it. (**c**) Excretory urogram fragments (a large additional cavity in the middle segment which was interpreted as a "cyst"). (**d**, **e**) Fragments of spot radiographs taken from the same patient in the vertical and horizontal positions (horizontal level of intensive contents in a spot upright image, an intensive rounded formation in the horizontal image)

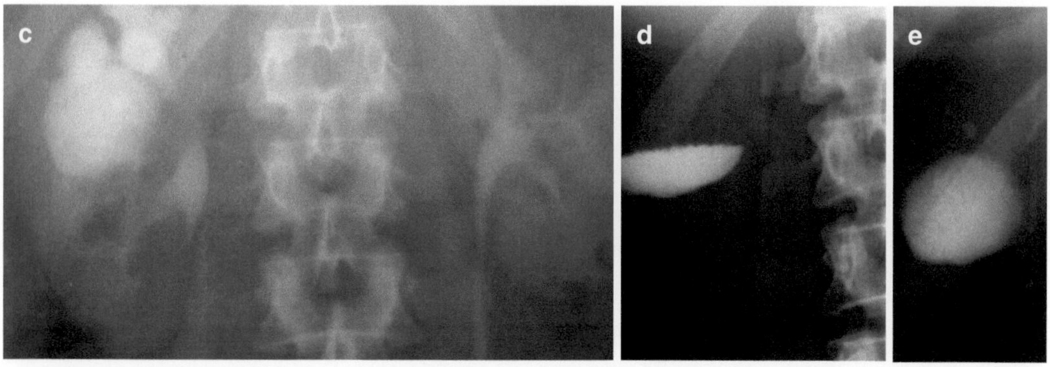

Fig. 1.30 (continued)

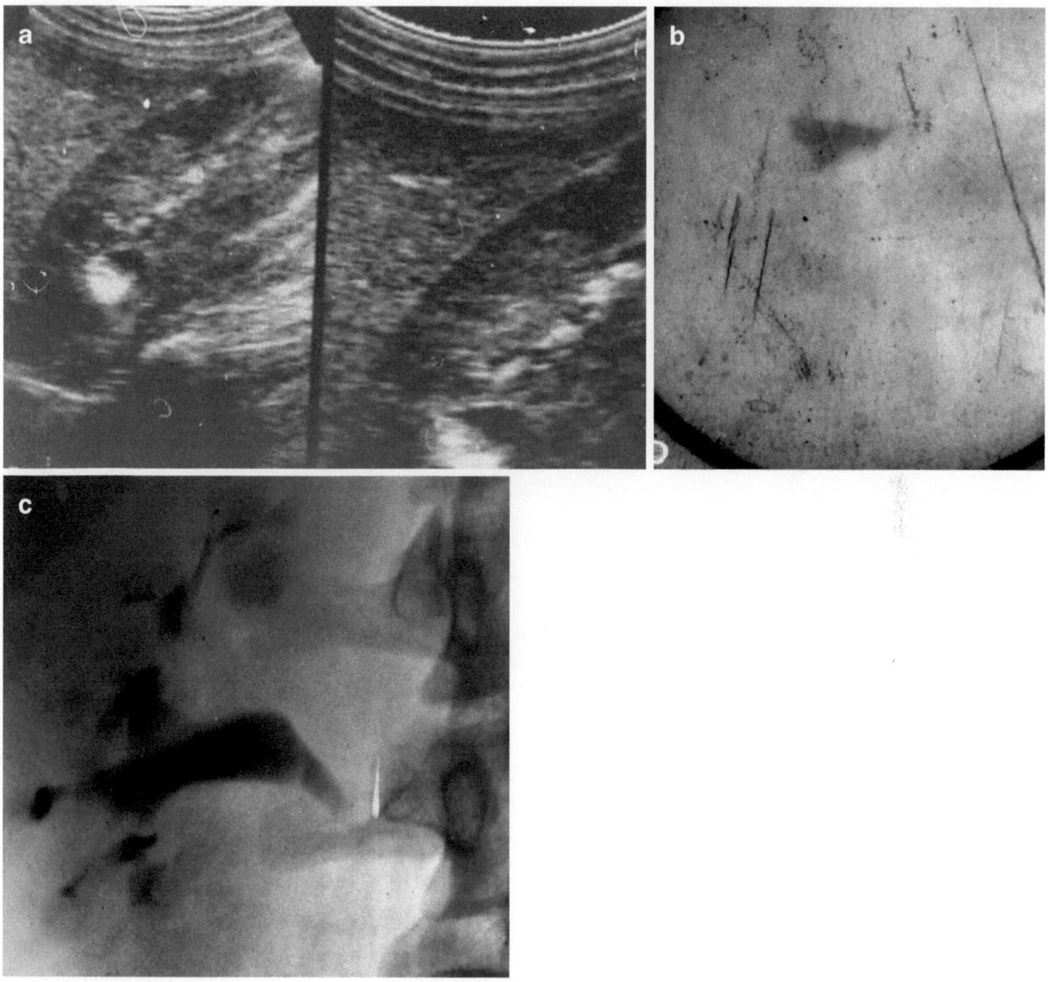

Fig. 1.31 A small diverticulum in an upper calyx of the right kidney with calcium milk: (**a**) in sonograms from patient lying on the right side; (**b**, **c**) in an overall spot radiogram and a fragment of excretory urogram, 15th min (a correct diagnosis was determined only after three inefficient RLs)

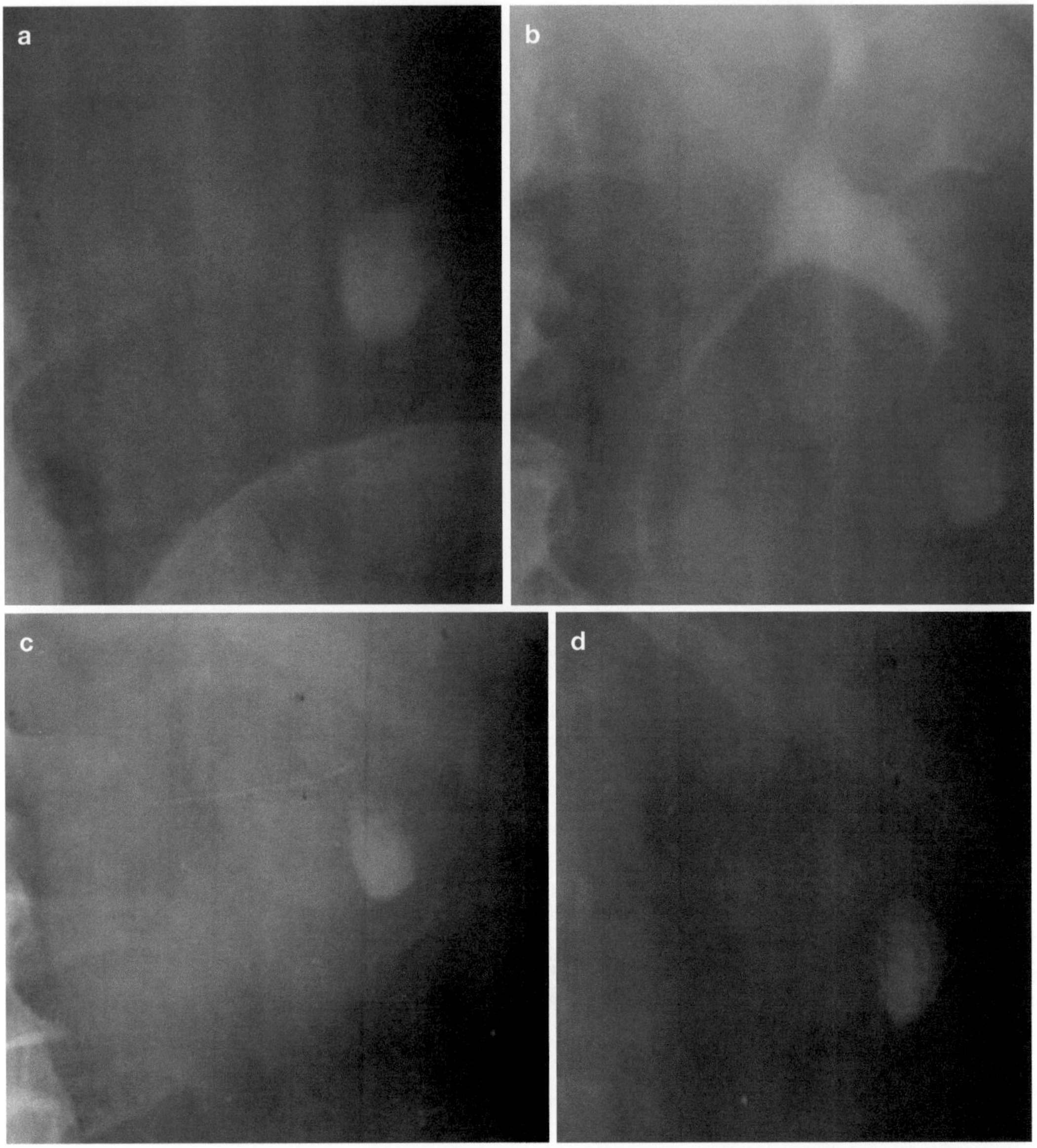

Fig. 1.32 (**a**) A fragment of an overall and (**b**) a fragment of excretory urogram, 15th min, with diverticulum in a lower calyx of the upper kidney (one seance of RL performed for a "stone" in a lower calyx). (**c–e**) Spot left kidney radiograms of the same female patient lying with face up and face down and in the vertical position—the "stone" is shifting in shape and forms a horizontal level when the patient is standing. (**f**) A typical ultrasound presentation of calyx diverticulum with a horizontal echo-producing level shifting along with the patient's posture which is formed by calcium milk (Data obtained by means of USG in a urological clinic)

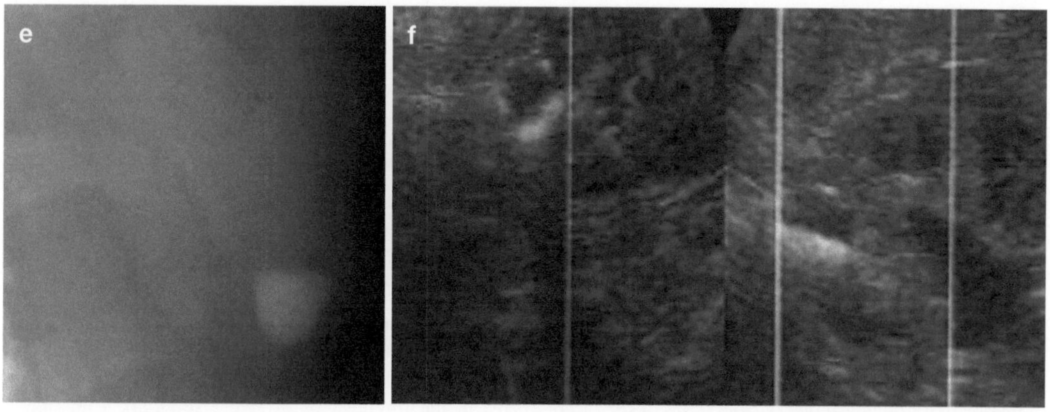

Fig. 1.32 (continued

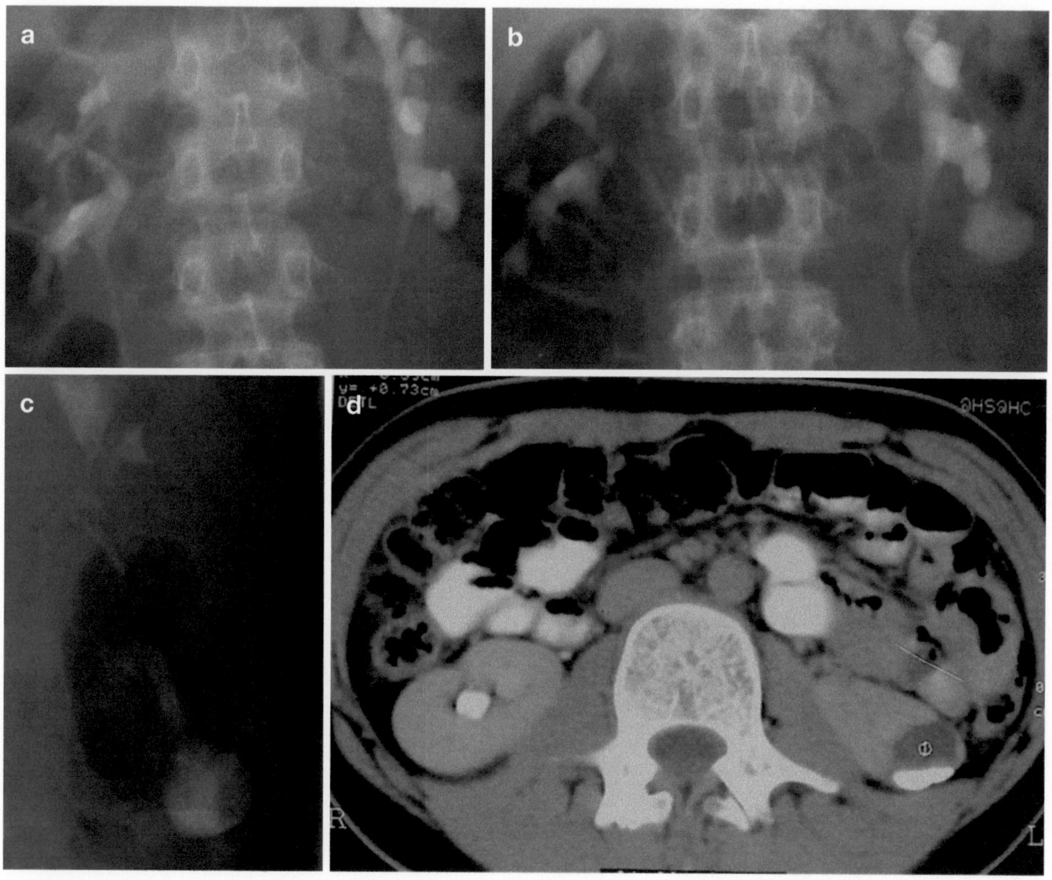

Fig. 1.33 (**a, b**) Growth of diverticulum in a lower calyx of the left kidney in three years; (**c**) calcium milk in the diverticulum in a lower calyx of the left kidney in spot delayed upright urograms; (**d**) a computer tomogram; the formation in the lower segment of the left kidney was interpreted as a cyst with "deposition" (differential diagnostics with the tuberculous caverna was performed)

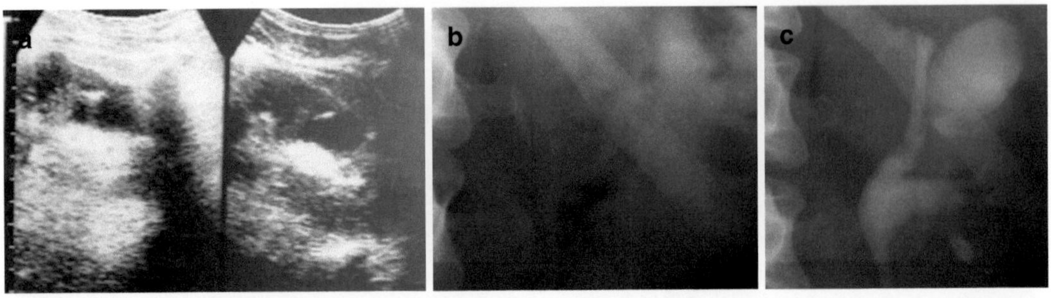

Fig. 1.34 An "accidental" discovery of a large diverticulum in an upper calyx with calcium milk in it (the female patient had a preclinical abdominal USG under program of treatment for duodenal ulcer): (**a**) a series of sonograms with an echo-free and echo-producing component which was interpreted as a "cyst with deposition" in the upper pole of the left kidney; (**b**) in the fragment of the overall radiogram of the left kidney, a shadow can be seen similar to a concrement in the upper segment of the left kidney; (**c**) in the fragment of excretory urogram, 15th min, a diverticulum in an upper calyx of the left kidney is observed

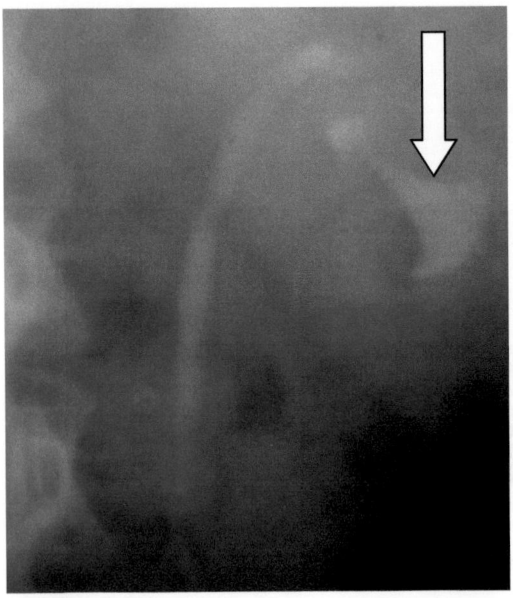

Fig. 1.35 A fragment of excretory urogram, congenital hydrocalycosis of the left kidney lower calyx (*arrow*)—a massive local dilatation of a lower calyx which has preserved its typical triangle shape

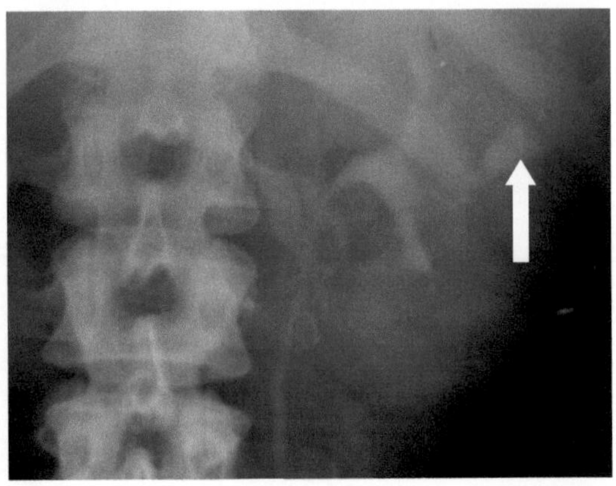

Fig. 1.36 A spot excretory urogram of the left kidney in case of acquired hydrocalycosis of a middle calyx (*arrow*)—dilatation of the middle calyx with its rounded expanded part and flattened fornix

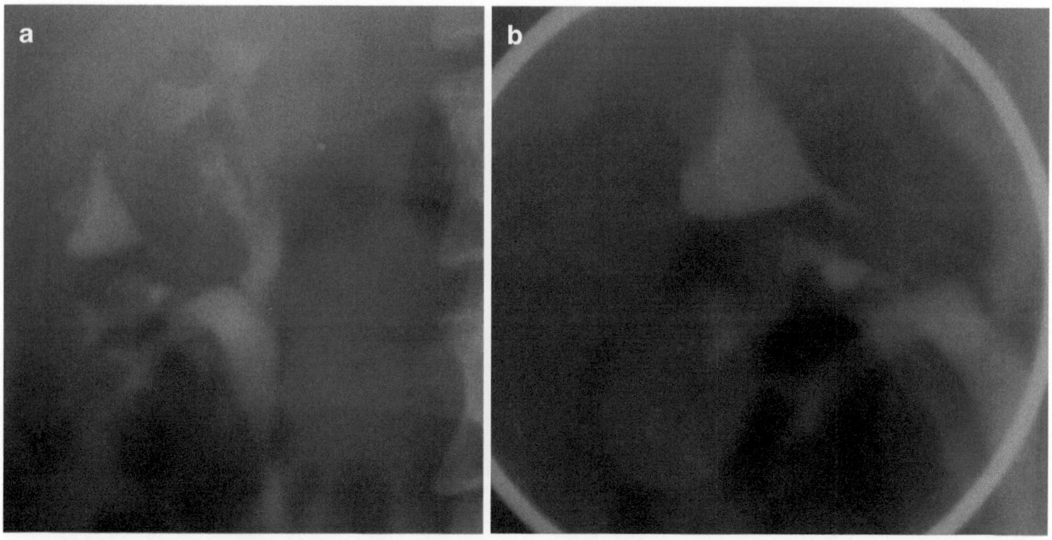

Fig. 1.37 Abnormality of pelvicalyceal system: detachment of an upper calyx and an additional middle calyx with hydrocalycosis and a small diverticulum (spontaneous stones expulsion in anamnesis); (**a**) in the excretory urogram, 15th min; (**b**) in a spot excretory urogram made under cineradiographic monitoring

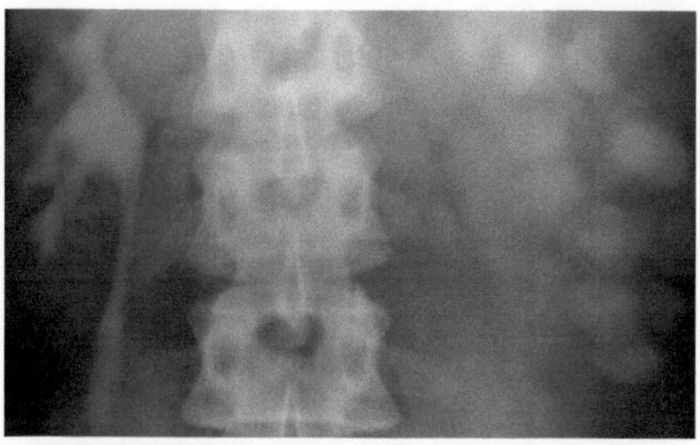

Fig. 1.38 Congenital megapolycalycosis of the left kidney, right ureter achalasia

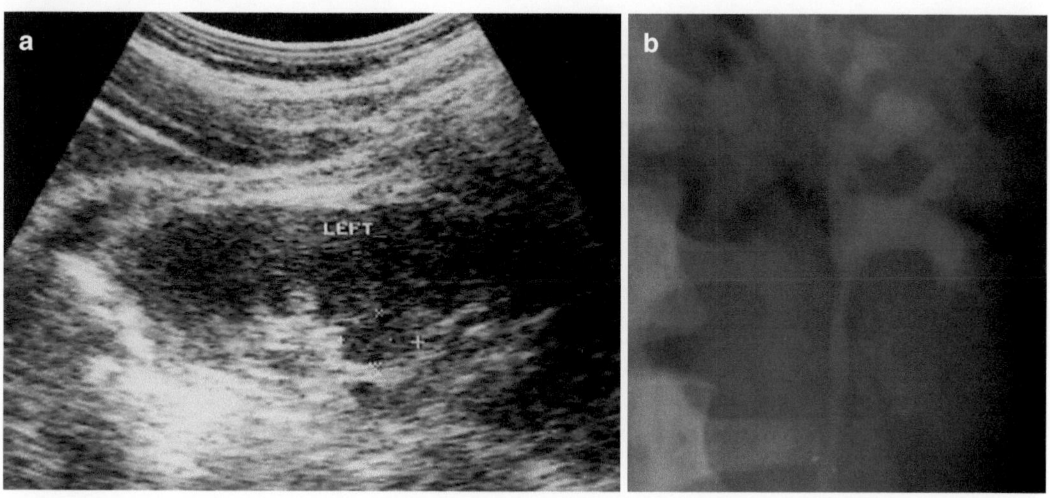

Fig. 1.39 (**a**, **b**) A sonogram and excretory urogram fragment—a congenital abnormality, namely, local hydrocalycosis of one of the upper calyces due to its "detachment," a kind of intrarenal doubling of the pelvicalyceal system

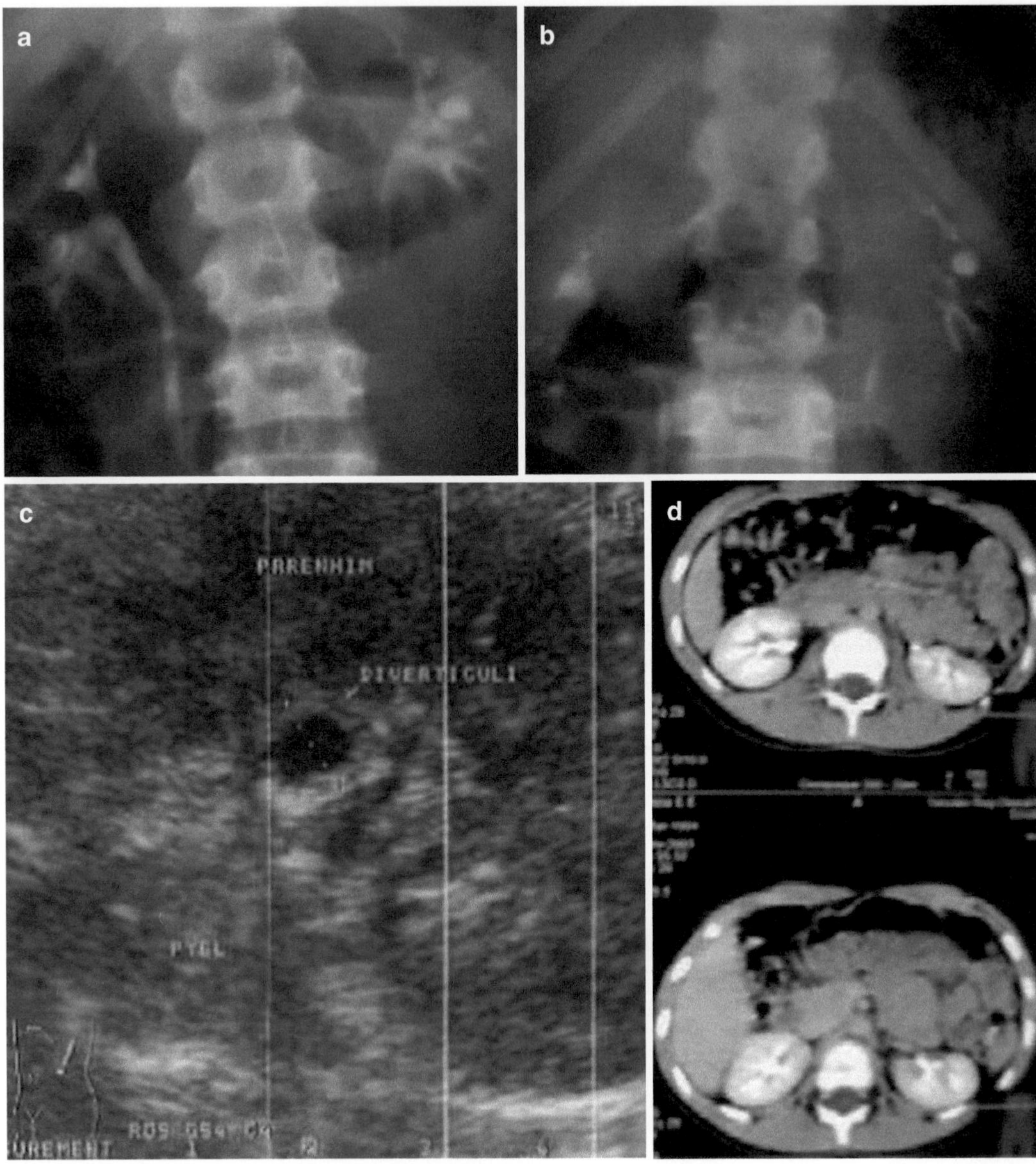

Fig. 1.40 (**a**, **b**) Excretory urograms in the 10th and 45th min of a female patient with diverticulum in an upper calyx of the left kidney who was getting treatment in a tuberculosis hospital for suspected cavernous tuberculosis of the left kidney (a rounded cavity in the fornical area of a middle calyx with intensiveness increase in a delayed image); (**c**, **d**) a sonogram and computer tomograms of the same patient (a small rounded echo-free formation in a cortical layer zero dynamics after a trial therapy with anti-tuberculosis medications)

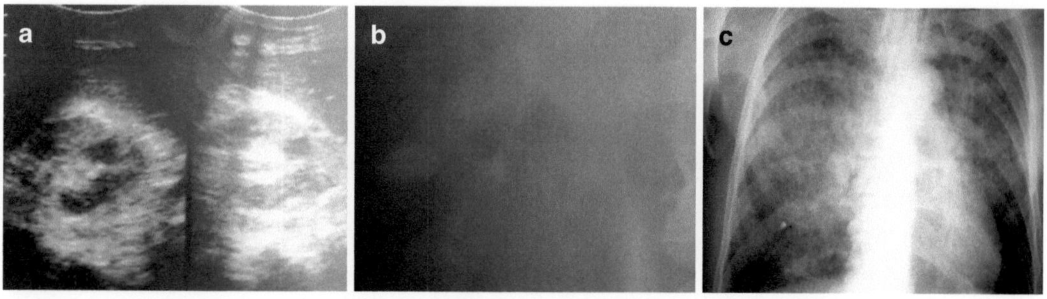

Fig. 1.41 A tuberculous cavern interpreted as a carbuncle of the right kidney middle segment; (**a**) sonogram, an echo-free formation in the parenchyma of the middle segment which was interpreted as a carbuncle; (**b**) a fragment of excretory urogram, 45th min, an additional cavity located to the medial side of a middle calyx and more intensively opacified in delayed images—middle calyx diverticulun or a tuberculous caverna (decapsulation and nephrostomy performed before nephrectomy on the right side); (**c**) a bilateral disseminated process in the lungs interpreted by the consultant phthisiologist as bilateral focal postoperative pneumonia. Tuberculous lesion of the right kidney detected in the course of histologic examination of the excised right kidney. The patient was transferred from urological clinic into tuberculosis hospital

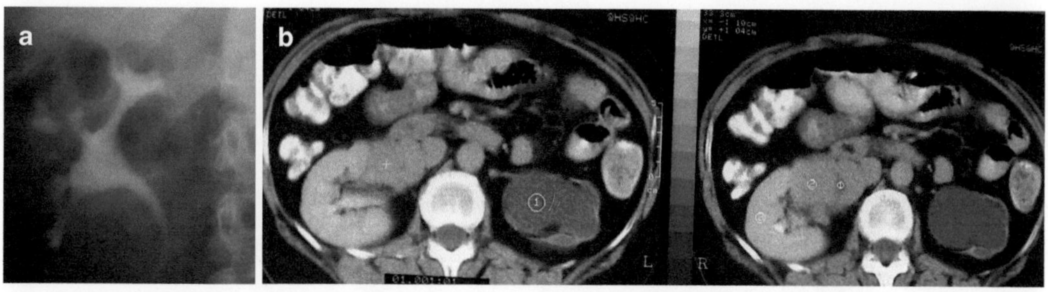

Fig. 1.42 Suspected tuberculous or diverticulum in a middle calyx of the upper kidney; (**a**) a fragment of excretory urogram, 10th min, an additional elongated asymmetric cavity connected with a middle calyx; (**b**) a series of computer tomograms—tumor of the lower segment of the right kidney and a hydronephrosis (nephropyosis) of the left kidney due to constriction of the lower left ureter of tubercular etiology The female patient refused surgery

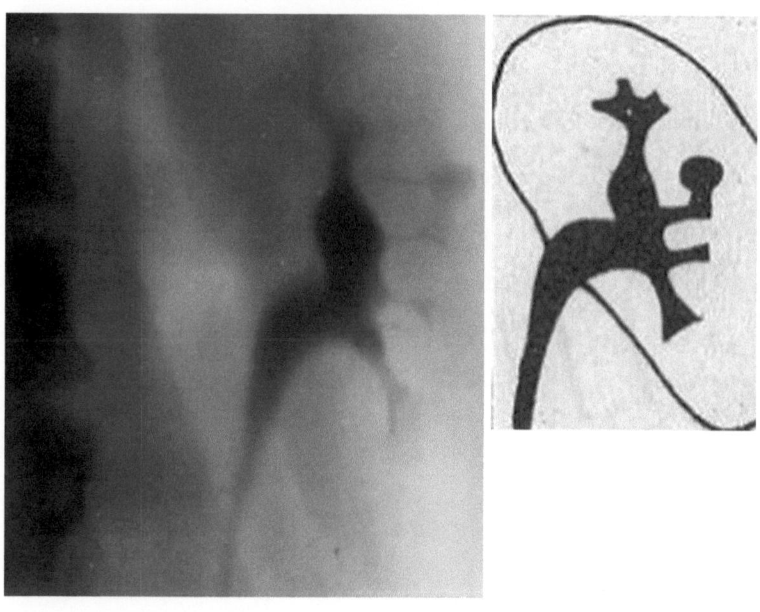

Fig. 1.43 Diverticulum in the middle calyx of the left kidney in an excretory urosonogram (EU) examination done for the left side renal colic which appeared for the first time in the patient's life; a tuberculous caverna was suspected (The first observation Perelman and Builov [22])

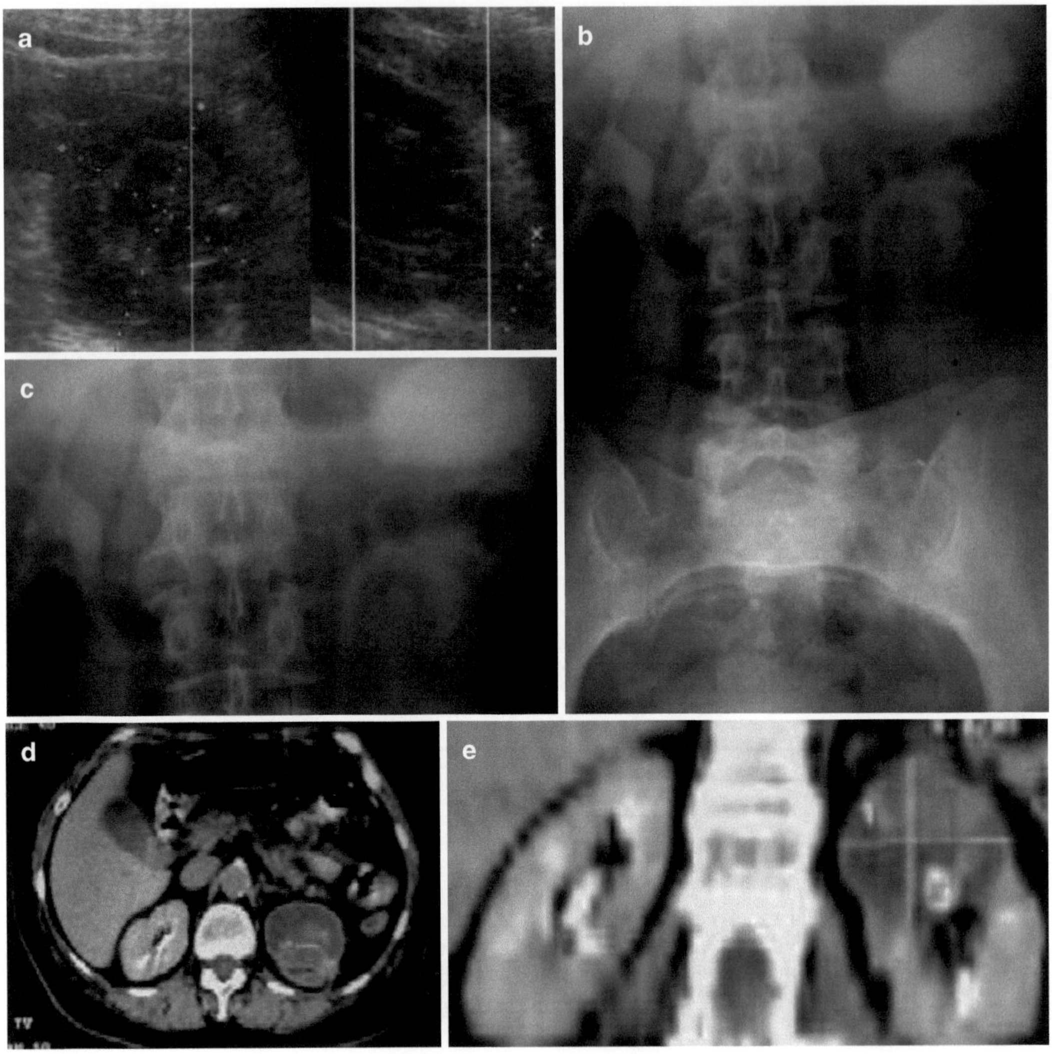

Fig. 1.44 Traumatic rupture of a cyst in the upper segment of the left kidney; its excretory urogram looked similar to a large diverticulum in an upper calyx, while USG and CAT simulated a renal tumor: (**a**) Formation in the upper segment of the left kidney with a complex echostructure which was interpreted during USG as a kidney tumor, in 2 days after trauma, accompanied by painless hematuria. (**b**, **c**) Excretory urograms in the 10th and 45th min taken from the same female patient on the 7th day after the trauma, which display a large cavity with sharp outlines in the upper segment of the left kidney; it has the same opacification like the pelvicalyceal system with increase in a delayed image and urographic presentation similar to a large diverticulum cavity in an upper calyx and not typical for a kidney tumor. (**d**, **e**) Computer tomograms of the same female patient in 10 days after the trauma, interpreted as a forming traumatic hematoma or a hemorrhage into a disintegrating kidney tumor. (**f**, **g**) A cyst of the upper kidney segment in a sonogram and excretory urogram in the same patient 12 years ago. (**h**) A formation on the upper segment of the left kidney which decreased from 5.0 to 1.5 cm in 1.5 month after the trauma

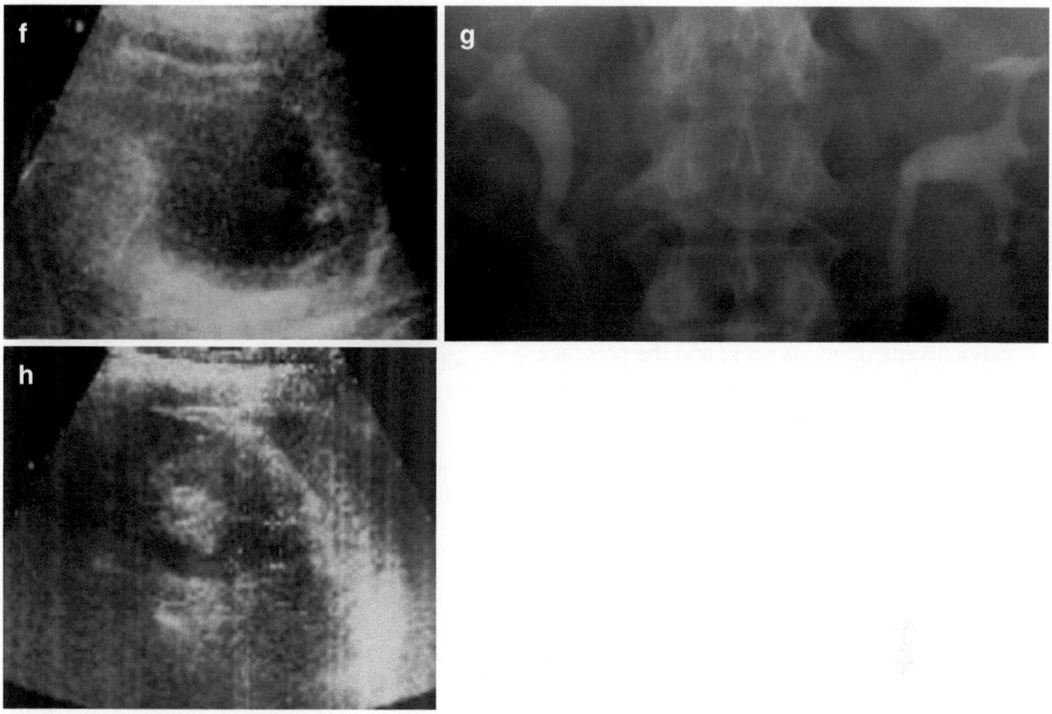

Fig. 1.44 (continued)

for the first time in order to determine its anatomical and topographic relations with the calyx diverticulum, magnetic resonance or excretory urography is recommended.

- In the absence of clinical presentations, ultrasound monitoring should be effected once every 1–2 years.

The algorithm for diagnostic imaging and selection of a treatment method for calyx diverticulum *complicated with calcium milk or lithogenesis is in our opinion as follows*:

- In case of a typical ultrasound presentation of a calyx diverticulum with calcium milk in it, a detection of horizontal level of highly opaque liquid in an upright spot X-ray image would be sufficient; RL and surgery are not recommended. Ultrasound monitoring once every 1–2 years is recommended.
- In case of a doubtful presentation of diverticulum with calcium milk or a suspected concrement in the diverticulum cavity, it is recommended to perform EU with multiple-view spot cineradiographic monitoring or SCTU with introduction of a normal dose of XRCM (*1.0 ml per 1.0 kg of patient's body weight, but no less than 40.0 ml of Ultravist, Omnipaque 300, or another non-ionic XRCM*) and a 3D image reconstruction in order to examine the diverticulum neck for the purpose of predicting the possibility of the stone fragment expulsion.
- In case of clinical response to the concrement, RL is recommended (with spontaneous stone fragment expulsion if possible) or surgical treatment, including endoscopic treatment.

Conclusion

In conclusion, we would like to emphasize the fact that semiology of calyx diverticulum imaging is rather typical and in most cases does not imply significant difficulties in differential diagnostics if specific knowledge and experience in calyx diverticulum diagnostics are present.

Ultrasound and X-ray examinations of a calyx diverticulum diagnostics, including the conventional spot or overall radiography as well as EU with the patient in horizontal and vertical positions, complemented with *cineradiographic monitoring of the upper urinary tract* and also the most efficient and state-of-the-art SCTU/MSCTU technologies all constitute a typical example of complementarity, not competition of the most commonly used methods of diagnostic imaging. This helps to obtain comprehensive information on the calyx diverticulum, its neck, and the presence of calcium milk or a concrement in its cavity which is the principal factor in selection of a treatment method.

Undoubtedly, a wider application of magnetic resonance urography will open new prospects in diagnostic imaging of pelvicalyceal system diverticula [98].

References

1. Rayer PP. Traite des maladies des reins. Urol. & Nephrol. 1841;3:507, Paris.
2. Pereverzev AS. Aspects of diagnostics and treatment of calyx diverticula. Issues Clin Exp Urol Nephrol. 1967;(1):153–156.
3. Pytel AY, Goligorodsky SD. Selected sections of nephrology and urology. Leningrad, Part 1, 1968.
4. Abeshouse BS, Abeshouse GA. Sponge kidney: a review of the literature and a report of five cases. J Urol (Baltimore). 1960;84:252–62.
5. Abeshouse BS, Abeshouse GA. Calyceal diverticulum: a report of 16 cases and review of the literature. Urol Intern. 1963;15:329–36.
6. Middleton AW, Pfiser RC. Stone-containing pyelocaliceal diverticulum: embryogenic, anatomic, radiologic and clinic characteristics. J Urol (Baltimore). 1974;111:2–6.
7. Topchan AB, Finkelstein SI. Roentgenologic atlas on urological diagnostics. Moscow: Medgiz; 1947.
8. Rutsky AV, Mihajlov AN. X-ray diagnostics atlas. Minsk: Vyshejshaya shkola; 1987, Part 2.
9. Pytel AY, Pugachyov AG. Essay on infantile urology. Moscow: Meditsina; 1977.
10. Pytel AY, Pytel YA. X-ray diagnostics of urological diseases. Moscow: Meditsina; 1961.
11. Tchuhrienko DP, Lyulko AV, Lukich VL. Roentgenological diagnostics of urological diseases. Moscow: Atlas; 1969.
12. Pytel YA. Classification of abnormalities of kidneys an urinary tract: materials of the 2-nd All-Union conference of urologists. Kiev, 1978.
13. Materials of the 2-nd All-Union conference of urologists. Urol Nephrol. 1979;1:3–9.
14. Karpenko VS, Pereverzev AS. Calyx diverticulum and solitary cyst– is it the same renal abnormality process? Materials of the 2-nd All-Union conference of urologists. Kiev, 1978.
15. Lopatkin NA, editor. Urology manual. Moscow: Meditsina; 1998.
16. Kumar S. Multiple ureteral diverticula. J Nat Med Ass. 1974;66:161–2 (Multiple ureteral diverticula. Russ Med J. 1975;1:18–19).
17. Golovko YI, et al. Paraureteral diverticulum and ureterocele in case of duplication of kidneys in children. Urol Nephrol. 1993;4:45–6.
18. Belmer SV, Gasilina TV. Comparison of uroexcretory and alimentary systems – morphofunctional and clinical parallels. Russ Med J. 2003;20:11–7.
19. Kottasz S, Hamvas A. Calyceal diverticulae. Int Urol Nephrol. 1976;8(3):203–12.
20. Lopatkin NA, Lylko AV. Abnormalities of urogenital system. Kiev: Zdorovja; 1987.
21. Dunnick NR, Sandler CM, Amis ES, Newhouse JH. Congenital anomalies in textbook of uroradiology. 2nd ed. Baltimore: Lippincott Williams & Wilkins; 1997.
22. Perelman VM, Builov VM. X-ray diagnostics of kidney diverticula. Bull Roentgenol Radiol. 1988;1:56–60.
23. Wulfsohn MA. Diagnosis and treatment of calyx diverticulae. J Urol. 1980;123:1–8.
24. Brunzema F. Die Klinische Bedeutung von Kalix-Zystem und pyelogenen Zystem im Hinblick auf ihre differential diagnostissche. Einordung Urologie Ausg. 1983;23:177–8.
25. Middleton AW, Pfiser RC. Stone-containing pyelocaliceal diverticulum: embryogenic, anatomic, radiologic and clinic characteristics. J Urol. 1974;111: 2–6.
26. Pytel YA, Zolotaryov II. Errors and complications at X-ray examination of kidneys and urinary tract. Moscow: Meditsina; 1987.
27. Amar AD. The clinical significance of renal caliceal diverticulum in children: relation to vesicoureteral reflux. J Urol. 1975;113:255–7.
28. Fraley EE. Vascular obstruction of superior infundibulum causing nephralgia: a new syndrome. New Engl J Med. 1966;275:1403–9.
29. Fraley EE. Surgical correction of intrarenal disease. J Urol. 1967;98:54–64.
30. Kumar S. Multiple ureteral diverticula. J Nat Med Ass. 1974;66:161–2 (Summary in the Russian language – multiple ureteral diverticula. Russ Med J. 1975;1:18).
31. Desgrez JP. Diverticulose ureterale. Ann Urol. 1983;17(2):96–8 (Summary in the Russian language. Russ Med J. 1983;19(10):14–5).
32. Masini G, Filli R, Vannucchi A. Stone of calyceal diverticulae. Radiol Med. 1980;66:509–12.
33. DeMarco RT, Cain MP, Davis MM. Xanthogranulomatous pyelonephritis associated with a congenital caliceal diverticulum. Urology. 2001;57(1): 168.
34. Garcia-Schurmann JM, Sommerfeld H, Pannek J. Spontaneous thrombosis of an iatrogenic arteriovenous fistula of the kidney. Urology. 2001;58(1):106.

35. Siegel MJ, McAlister WH. Calyx divertuculae in children: unusual futures and complications. Radiology. 1979;131:79–82.
36. Akyaev YG, Amosov AV, Krapivin AA, et al. Spontaneous kidney rupture. Sono Ace Int. 2006;14:3–8. Russian version.
37. Rudstroem P. Hydrocalyx. Acta Chir Scand. 1949;98: 34–9.
38. Garrett RA, Holland JM. Milk-of-calcium in caliceal diverticulum. J Urol (Baltimore). 1967;109:927–9.
39. Healey T, Way BG, Grind WR. Milk of calcium in calyx diverticulae. Brit J Radiol. 1980;56(3):845.
40. Builov VM, Karpov NR, Aliferov BD, et al. Ultrasound and X-ray diagnostics for selecting a method of treatment for calcium milk and stones: materials of conference of the Yaroslavl region medical and pharmaceutical professionals. St. Petersburg Part 2, 2003.
41. Builov VM, Karpov NR, Aliferov BD. 15-year experience in sound and X-ray diagnostics of kidney diverticula. St. Petersburg: Materials of the Neva Radiological Forum; 2005.
42. Seung Hyup KIM, editor. Radiology illustrated: uroradiology. Philadelphia: Sanders; 2003.
43. Builov VM. Symptoms of calcium milk, rattlebox and twinking artifact in ultrasound and X-ray diagnostics of calyx diverticula prior to remote lithotripsy: abstracts of reports of the anniversary interregional science and practice conference on modern approaches to urolithiasis treatment in adults and children. 9–10 Feb 2006. Yaroslavl, 2006.
44. Hitrova AN, Mitkov VV, Mitkova MD. Ultrasound diagnostics of kidney diseases: practical guide to ultrasound diagnostics. Moscow: VIDAR Publishing House; 2005, under editorship of Mitkova VV.
45. Builov VM, Turzin VV, Carpov NR. Ultrasound diagnosis of calyceal diverticulum: 4th European symposium on uroradiology. 12–15 Sept. Florence, 1994.
46. Builov VM, Turzin VV, Karpov NR. Sonographic diagnostics of calyx diverticula. Vis Clin. 1993;3(1):21–3.
47. Builov VM. Combined application and algorithms of ultrasound и scanning and X-ray diagnostics of renal and ureteral diseases: abstract of thesis… doctor of medicine. Moscow, 1994.
48. Gromov AI, Kubova SY. Clinical significance of Doppler twinking artifact detection at ultrasound examination of internal organs. St. Petersburg: Materials of the 2nd International Congress of the Neva Radiological Forum; 2005:34–35 .
49. Demidov VN, Pytel YA, Amosov AV. Ultrasound diagnostics in uronephrology. Moscow: Meditsina; 1989. p. 54.
50. Amosov AV, Imnaishvili GI. Pharmacosonography: materials of the 8-th All-Russia conference of urologists. Moscow, 1988.
51. Bilgasem S, Pace KT, Dyer S, Honey RJ. Erect and supine radiographs to assess effectiveness of SWL for stones in a caliceal diverticulum or dilated calix. J Endourol. 2003;17(1):7–9.
52. Kavukcu S, Cakmakci H, Babayigit A. Diagnosis of caliceal diverticulum in two pediatric patients: a comparison of sonography, CT and urography. J Clin Ultrasound. 2003;31(4):218–21.
53. Wulfsohn MA. Intravenous urography in diagnosis of calyceal diverticula. J Urol. 1980;123:1–8.
54. Builov VM. Ultrasound and X-ray diagnostics of pelvicalyceal diverticula. Sono Ace Int. 2006;14:9–19. Russian version.
55. Ternovoj SK, Alyaev YG, Sinitsyn VE, et al. Diagnostic capabilities and clinical application of magnetic-resonance urography. Med Vis. 2001;2:72–7.
56. Alyaev YG, Sinitsyn VE, Grigoriev NA. Magnetic resonance imaging in urology. Moscow: Prakticheskaya Meditsina; 2005.
57. Dombrovsky VI. Magnetic-resonance imaging in diagnostics of tumour and other diseases of kidneys. MRI-pathoanatomy comparison: Atlas. Moscow: VIDAR Publishing House; 2003.
58. Neri E, Borashi P, Caramella D, et al. MR virtual endoscopy of the upper urinary tract. AJR. 2000; 175:1697–702.
59. Nolte-Ernsting CCA, Adam GB, Gunter RW. MR urography: examination techniques and clinical application. Eur Radiol. 2001;11:355–72.
60. Nolte-Ernsting CCA, Staatz G, Tacke J, et al. MR urography today. Abdom Imaging. 2003;28(2): 191–209.
61. Borthne A, Pierre-Jerome C, Nordshus T, et al. MR-urography in children current status and future development. Eur Radiol. 2000;10:503–11.
62. Jung P, Brauers A, Notle-Ernsting CA, et al. Magnetic resonance urography enhanced by gadolinium and diuretics: a comparison with conventional urography in diagnosing the cause of ureteric obstruction. BJU Int. 2000;86:960–5.
63. El-Diasty T, Mangour O, Furoux A. Diuretic contrast-enhanced magnetic resonance urography versus intravenous urography for depiction of nondilated urinary tracts. Abdom Imaging. 2003;29:135–95.
64. Pytel YA, Zolotaryov II. On diagnostic errors in case of retentional calyx changes. Urol Nephrol. 1974;4: 23–9.
65. Rosenfield AT, Richman T. The urinary tract. Atlas of ultrasonography, vol. 2. New York/Edinburgh/London/Melbourne: Churchill Livingstone; 1985. p. 891–3.
66. Pilipenko NV, Nazarenko VA. Ultrasound diagnostics in urology. Moscow: St. Petersburg; 1993.
67. Karpenko VS, Pereverzev AS. Megacalicosis. Vrachebnoye Delo. 1975;5:66–9.
68. Kulakov GP, Perelman VM. On detection of medullar sponge kidney. Radiol Diagn. 1970;11(2):227–35.
69. Kasaev AA, Simonenko AL. On X-ray diagnostics of sponge kidney in children. Bull Roentgenol Radiol. 1981;3:73–4.
70. Grund VD, Voskresensky BN. Overdiagnostics of nephrotuberculosis: quantitative and qualitative error analysis in patients with kidney abnormalities: theses of the 8-th All-Russia conference of urologists. Moscow, 1982.
71. Shabad AL. Nephrotuberculosis. Tashkent: Meditsina; 1978. p. 98.

72. Voskresensky BN. Tuberculosis and congenital abnormalities of kidneys: abstract of thesis… candidate of medical science. Moscow, 1982.
73. Grund VD, Voskresensky BN. Differential diagnostics of tuberculous caverna and calyx diverticulum. Urol Nephrol. 1983;1:8–13.
74. Morozov NV. Megacalycosis as the cause of nephrotuberculosis overdiagnostics. Bull Roentgenol Radiol. 1985;6:86–7.
75. Gagarinov VS. Diagnostics of rare abnormalities of renal development and structure. Bull Roentgenol Radiol. 1979;2:29–34.
76. Olsson O. In: Handbuch der Urologie. Berlin: St. Petersburg; 1962. p. 92–97.
77. Grund VD. Errors in diagnostics and treatment of tuberculosis of urinary organs, vol. 1. Moscow: Meditsine; 1975. p. 25–40.
78. Kamyshan IS, Sejmivsky DA, Gagarinov VS, et al. Rare renal structure abnormalities simulating tuberculosis: materials of the 2-nd All-Union conference of urologists. Kiev, 1978.
79. Borisov VV, Shapiro AL. Specific aspects of X-ray diagnostics of nephrotuberculosis. Bull Roentgenol Radiol. 1976;4:49–53.
80. Zbang JO, Fielding JR, Zou KH, et al. Etiology of spontaneous perirenal hemorrhage: a meta-analysis. J Urol. 2002;167:1593–6.
81. Abdelwahab A, Coloby P, Elias E. Laparoscopic treatment of symptomatic calculus diverticulum of the calyx. Prog Urol. 2001;11(4):752–6.
82. Munver R, Delvecchio FC, Newman GE, Preminger GM. Critical analysis of supracostal access for percutaneous renal surgery. J Urol. 2001;166(4):1242–6.
83. Wolf Jr JS. Caliceal diverticulum and hydrocalyx. Laparoscopic management. Urol Clin North Am. 2000;27(4):655–60.
84. Lancini V, Liatsikos EN, Bernardo NO, et al. Percutaneous treatment of calculosis in caliceal diverticulosis: 13-year experience. Arch Ital Urol Androl. 2000;72(2):59–63.
85. Al-Basam S, Bennett JD, Layton ZA, et al. Treatment of caliceal diverticular stones: transdiverticular percutaneous nephrolithotomy with creation of a neoinfundibulum. J Vasc Interv Radiol. 2000;11(7):885–9.
86. Curran MJ, Little AF, Bouyounes B, et al. 3rd experience retroperitoneoscopic technique for treating symptomatic caliceal diverticula. J Endourol. 1999;13(10):723–5.
87. Landry JL, Colombel M, Rouviere O, et al. Long term results of percutaneous treatment of caliceal diverticular calculi. Eur Urol. 2002;41(4):474–7.
88. Miller SD, Ng CS, Streem SB, Gill IS. Laparoscopic management of caliceal diverticular calculi. J Urol. 2002;167(3):1248–52.
89. Torrecilla OC, Colom FS, Contreras GJ, et al. Current treatment of lithiasis in congenital renoureteral malformations. Arch Esp Urol. 2001;54(9):926–36.
90. Gaur DD. Retroperitoneal laparoscopic ureterolithotomy. World J Urol Nephrol. 1993;27:75–6.
91. Andersson T. The radilogist's role during the endourology procedures: 10th European symposium on urogenital radiology. 4–7 Sept. Sweden, 2003.
92. Kikuchi E, Sumitomo M, Hatakeyama N, et al. Percutaneous endoscopic marsupialization of a pyelocaliceal diverticulum with milk of calcium stones. Tokyo: Department of Urology, Keio University School of Medicine; 1998.
93. Builov VM, Smolyakov YB, Patrunov YN. Ultrasound and X-ray diagnostics for selecting a treatment program for stones in calyx diverticula. Urology. 2006;4:61–5.
94. Builov VM. Diagnostic imaging of pelvicalyceal system diverticula. Moscow: Vidar; 2007, 94 with illustrations.
95. Smith A. Treatmen of *calyx diverticula*, the first Russian congress of endourologists. 4–6 June 2008, Moscow. http://www.uro.ru/meetings/1447html.
96. Builov VM. Ultrasound and X-ray diagnostics of traumatic and iatrogenic damage of renal cyst walls. Sonoace Ultrasound Issue Moscow 20, 2010, p. 83–88.
97. Builov VM. Algorithm of uroradiological diagnostics in 2010 medical visualisation. Special issue 2010 materials of the 4th All-Russian National Congress of ray diagnostics and therapists. Radiology. Moscow, 25–27 May 2010, p. 65–6.
98. Builov VM. An experience of low field magnetic resonance visualization by means of an open MRI unit in urology. Diagnostic and interventional radiology. Crossdiscip Sci Prac J. 2011;5(2):77, Supplement, Materials of the 5th All-Russia National Congress of ray diagnostics and therapy *Radiology 2011*, Moscow, 25–27 May 2011.

2 Diagnostics of Ureteral Diverticula

Ureteral diverticulum (UD) is a saccular outpouching of the ureteral wall which may vary in size and location. Diverticulum wall consists of the same layers as the ureter. The inner surface of UD is covered with urothelium; the submucosal layer is usually subtle. In the embryologic aspect, UD are additional outpouchings of the caudal end of the coelenteron, and they develop as an additional ureter anlage. UD can be found in any part of the ureter, on one or both sides, but the most frequent location is the pelvic area, more often on the right.

UD, the same as diverticula of any other part of the urinary tract, are divided into *congenital and acquired ones*. According to some authors, UD is mostly of *acquired* nature and is related with ureter diminution caused by various traumas or by consequences of surgeries or resulting from ureter wall decubitus formed under a concrement and followed by an infection which weakens the ureter wall and provokes UD formation [1–3].

Congenital UD are observed very rarely and are usually discovered accidentally. Harlin and Atkinson [4] found only 18 descriptions of congenital UD in the literature and added an observation of their own. Desgrez [5], who described UD in the lower part of the right ureter in 1983, considered his observation to be the 26th case in the global literature. Sparsity of UD is also confirmed by statistics from the Mayo Clinic (1977) [6], where only 12 UD cases were discovered for 25 years (they are not divided into congenital and acquired in the report), and by statistics from the urological 100-bed clinic Perm Medical Academy (2008) [7], where for the same period, 25 years, only one patient was diagnosed with ureteral diverticulum among the 766 patients with ureteral abnormalities, while the latest publication on a congenital UD issued in 2005 is only the third one in the Japanese literature [8].

The first publication in the domestic literature devoted to demonstration of a hydronephrosis preparation containing a ureteral diverticulum (UD) was made by N. V. Sklifosovsky, an outstanding Russian surgeon [9].

From time to time, individual personal observations of UD are reported in the domestic and overseas literature which are supplemented by various statistical reference data, from singular cases to dozens of descriptions collected by various authors [3, 8, 10–40].

According to Culp [41], the specific sign of UD which is considered a rare congenital abnormality is the presence of a saccular outpouching of the ureter wall. This protrudes at an angle from the main ureter and maintains the minute structure typical for the ureter. UD length always exceeds its double diameter. The author observed three girls (4, 11, and 13 years old) with UD. No specific signs of UD were found. All the patients had the clinical presentation of chronic pyelonephritis. UD can be treated only by surgical methods. One patient had nephroureterectomy; the others had UD resection. All UD contained cloudy urine. Histologic examination revealed UD wall structure identical to the ureter structure with signs of inflammatory infiltration.

V.M. Builov, *Imaging of Urinary Tract Diverticula*,
DOI 10.1007/978-3-319-05383-7_2, © Springer International Publishing Switzerland 2014

According to Delmas and Delmas [10] UD are often discovered incidentally. The author described a 77-year-old patient who had multiple UD on the left in the pelvic area, while the upstream parts of the upper urinary tract remained unchanged. These diverticula were "accidentally" discovered when the patient was examined for painless intensive macrohematuria which had developed due to overdose of blood thinners. Based on that observation and 30 more UD cases collected from the reference literature, it is considered that UD, including multiple ones, are usually discovered incidentally. In men UD were found more often (22 observations), and about half of the patients had bilateral UD (16 observations). Deranged urodynamics in the upper urinary tract was discovered in 15 patients, and 9 patients had urinary tract infections

There is a description of an incidental UD finding which was made during examination of children with recurrent urinary tract infections. 17 UD are described including 14 pediatric patients. All patients had VUR which was complicated with recurrent urinary infections in 13 patients, with various dysuric phenomena in 3 patients, with enuresis in 2 patients, and with macrohematuria in 2 patients. Thirteen patients had retentional changes on UD side. The main reason for X-ray examination was VUR, while the discovered UD were, according to the authors, an "incidental finding" [29, 30]. These authors emphasize the fact that in descriptions by other authors, VUR is mentioned as a very rare phenomenon which accompanies UD and facilitates its diagnostics.

Sparsity of UD is confirmed by observation of six patients: two patients had UD on the left and four on the right. One patient was suspected to have an ovarian cyst. Another female patient had a necessary nephrectomy due to purulent pyelonephritis which developed after diverticulectomy and ureteroneocystostomy [27].

Aivazyan A.V. and Vojno-Yasenetsky A.M. in their review of literature on UD provide data that in 1936 Brown collected 9 descriptions of congenital UD from the literature, in 1950 Harlin and Atkinson collected as many as 18 descriptions of congenital UD and added one of their own (a 56-year-old male), and in 1959 Stachler discovered 13 more observations of this kind [28].

One of the authors [15] described his observation of a 5-year-old boy with a 5.0×3.0 cm UD who finally had the diverticulum Resection. Six months after the surgery, function of the kidneys was unchanged. Ectasia of the ureter up to 1.5 cm along 5–6 cm of the pelvic part over the area of UD resection still remained.

UD, the same as diverticula of any other part of the urinary tract, are divided into *congenital and acquired ones. Congenital ureteral diverticula* are observed in extremely rare cases. In ureterograms they look like ureteral wall outpouchings, and since this congenital abnormality is usually related with irregularity of urine passage down from the upper urinary tract, it may be combined with hydronephrosis and hydroureter. Congenital UD are usually small. In the literature only a few cases of large diverticula observations are described [3]. Diverticulum may appear in any part of the ureter.

Congenital ureteral diverticulum is rather a rare abnormality of the urinary tract. In report [30] only 15 cases out of 52 were classified as congenital. In majority of patients clinical presentations appear as late as above 20 years old and are as follows: pains and urinary tract infections; in some cases, there is a palpable formation which causes various diagnostic errors.

Congenital UD results from disturbances of embryogenesis of the urogenital system. Some researchers regard congenital UD as an incomplete double ureter. That is, a blind-ended branch of the ureter formed at its incomplete duplication, a kind of ureter appendage which can spring at any level.

In the Russian literature [18], a 24-year-old female patient is described (13-year catamnesis) who was urgently operated on for a twisted cyst of the left ovary which was not found. One month later she was admitted to the gynecology department again and diagnosed with acute parametritis and 16-week pregnancy. The second surgery was performed in the urology department with preoperatively diagnosed hydronephrosis on the third accessory kidney on the left (which contained

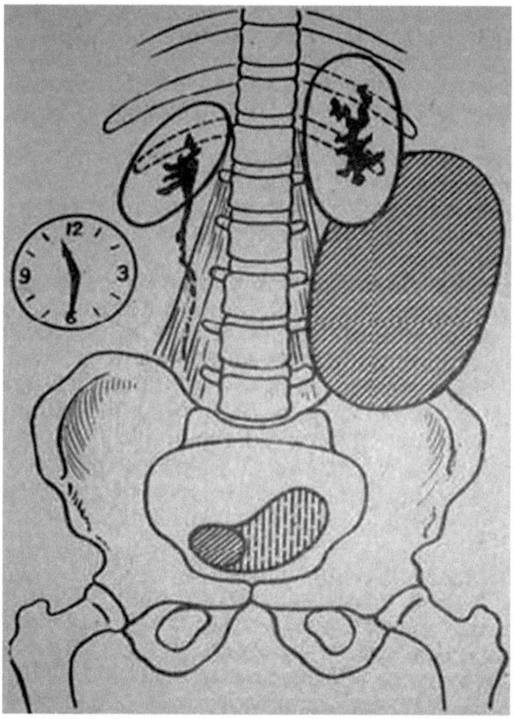

Fig. 2.1 A schematic drawing of excretory urogram made prior to the surgery (After Rzheznikov [19])

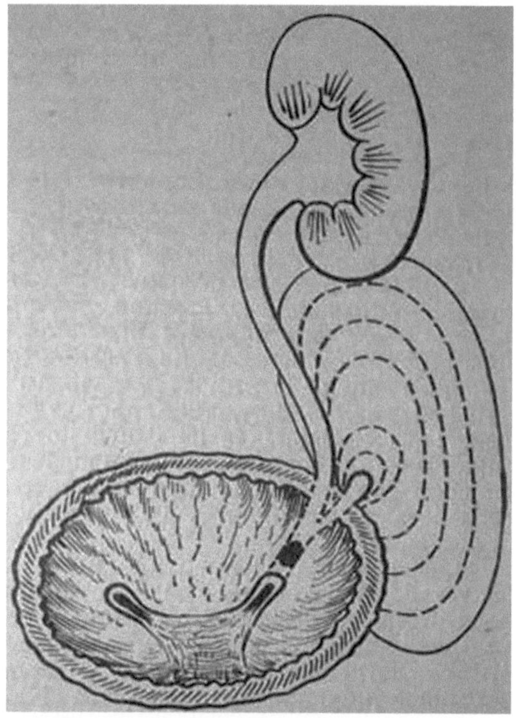

Fig. 2.2 Scheme of growth of a tumor like cystous formation (After Rzheznikov [19])

1.5 l of urine). The patient was operated on by A. Ya. Pytel who carried out ureterocystoneostomy. The removed preparation contained no layers which would be typical for the ureter wall, but the author explained it by UD expansion from 1.0 cm in diameter to a gigantic stretched bag where granulation tissue with cicatrization started to prevail due to a prolonged inflammatory process (Figs. 2.1 and 2.2).

As Aivazyan and Vojno-Yasenetsky note [28], congenital ureteral diverticulum is a shallow formation which is nearly always located in the pelvic area of the ureter and is connected with its lumen by means of a more or less wide duct. UD may have various shapes (round, ovoid, saccular, irregular, tubulous, etc.). UD usually has a small capacity, from 3 to 15 ml. UD wall structure vaguely resembles the structure of the ureter wall. UD usually has urothelial lining and a muscular layer, but in most cases urothelial cells are subject to metaplasia, and often they have pseudopolypous proliferations; the structure of muscular layers is irregular, and sometimes only individual muscular fibers are found which are located among the coarse fibrous tissue.

True UD (unlike blind-ended branches of accessory ureter) are not necessarily related with duplication or divarication of the ureter. In many cases UD are multiple and bilateral. Parts of the ureter which are located above UD, as well as the pelvicalyceal system and the kidney, are developed properly; sometimes more or less prominent secondary retentional changes are present.

Aivazyan and Vojno-Yasenetsky [28] classify UD as a congenital abnormality of the 1st clinical and functional type (congenital abnormalities which do not require treatment). Complications and concomitant diseases are very rare in the case of UD. This makes the theory of their acquired nature [18] caused by congenital or acquired diseases unpersuasive. Pytel and Tchebanyuk [37] suppose that "the diverticulum develops as an accessory ureter anlage." In the opinion of Aivazyan and Vojno-Yasenetsky [28], the most probable explanation is the following: the blind-ended accessory ureter of UD at various stages of their embryo morphogenesis is a divaricated branch of the metanephric duct which stopped to develop. In case an accessory ureter forms, the development stops later when a structure identical with the normal ureter is completed but has a blind end. In case of UD divarication is not followed by further growth; thus, a saccular formation appears which is connected with the main ureter and bears signs of histogenetic affinity to the ureter (urothelial lining, muscular layer), but its structure is not at all similar to a normal or blind-ended ureter. In the opinion of most researchers [27–30], the congenital UD is a duplex ureter which has an inlet and outlet leg or a blind-ended ureter branch. UD development may be stimulated by concurrent infections, reflux, and presence of stones. UD formation is caused by an abnormality of the ureter area where autonomic ganglions are absent, but there is a prominent rugosity of the mucosa which disturbs urodynamics.

As noted by Pytel and Pytel [38], in case two ureters are discovered on one side and one of them is blind ended, it must be kept in mind that the same presentation can be observed in case of a ureteral diverticulum (UD). According to Pytel and Pytel [38], UD is mostly of *acquired nature* and is related with ureter diminution caused by various traumas or by consequences of surgeries or resulting from ureter wall decubitus formed under a concrement.

The hypothesis of acquired UD nature also has it that UD develops due to *overlay of infectious process and obstructed urine drainage*. The infectious inflammatory process weakens the ureteral wall in some areas, and high pressure of urine provokes diverticula formation.

As mentioned above, UD is classified as a rare abnormality which consists of the formation of a saccular outpouching in the ureteral wall that may have various size and location but is mostly located on the right and in the pelvic area of the ureter. Extremely rare UD is found in the ureter area near the renal pelvis. Bilateral UD are also described. Hyperinflated UD constricts the adjacent part of the ureter, causing its obstruction with respective clinical presentations. Ureteral diverticulum has the same complications as calyx diverticulum: inflammation, lithogenesis, ureteropyelocaliectasis, and perforation.

True UD (different from blind-ended branches of accessory ureter) are not necessarily related with ureter duplication or divarication. UD are often multiple or bilateral. Parts of the ureter which are located above UD, as well as the pelvicalyceal system and the kidney, are developed properly; sometimes more or less prominent secondary retentional changes are present. Three patients are described [28] with small (up to 2–3 cm) solitary UD in the perivesical part of the ureter which had ovoid shape and were connected with the ureteral lumen by a narrow duct; no retentional changes of the UUT were present. All UD were "accidental" findings made during examinations for hematuria, enuresis, and proteinuria. No indications for surgical treatment of UD were found.

The majority of authors, as emphasized in Aivazyan and Vojno-Yasenetsky [28], also believe that diverticulectomy and resection of the perivesical part of the ureter in combination with ureterocystoneoanastomosis are justified only in rare cases, when UD has unusually big size, lithogenesis is present, or there are prominent disturbances of urodynamics on the UD side.

Excretory urography is the main method of UD diagnostics. Excretory urograms display a globular or saccular accessory cavern which has a sharp outline and is directly adjoining the ureter, the ureter being constricted in that area. The rate of the contrast medium accumulation in the cavity of the UD increases on delayed images, while UD opacification persists after the contrast medium discharge from the upper urinary tract.

As emphasized by [28, 38], the main method of UD diagnostics is X-ray examination. If the kidneys' function is satisfactory, usually the boundary of the ureter and its diverticulum is clearly seen in excretory urograms all over the ureter length. The authors explain these presentations by the pendulent ureteroureteral reflux (PUR) at the point of the UD divarication. At a diminished function of the kidneys, the authors used cystography: If PUR was present, the contrast medium filled both the ureter and its diverticulum. If PUR was absent, diagnostics were made by means of *retrograde ureteropyelography* which permitted to define the exact location and size of the diverticulum as well as the spot of its divarication from the main ureter.

In retrograde ureterograms UD are often diagnosed as strictures since the diverticulum neck is narrowed and, therefore, it may be difficult to achieve a good diverticulum filling with the contrast medium. It is not always possible to opacify the UD cavity during retrograde urography because of its inlet narrowing or the presence of a concrement; that's why in many cases UD are discovered only during a surgery [14, 19].

The only illustration present in the domestic literature is the one in the work by Lopatkin and Lyulko [39] which in turn was copied from a work by Desgrez [5] who described the 26th observation of UD. A 73-year-old woman was admitted for examination for recurrent cystitis. The cystitis recurred about two times a year and was relieved efficiently by short-term usage of antibiotics. Microhematuria persisted in the patient, and due to that reason, EU was performed. A specific image of the lumbar part of the left ureter was discovered which looked like a bunch of grapes. UD was described for the first time in 1957 (Holly and Sumead). Based on the analysis of the data from the literature and the abovementioned observation, it is emphasized that UD is found mostly in men aged 23–85 years old. No similar observations in children have been reported up to the moment. Twelve patients had bilateral UD, 11 patients had UD on the left, and 3 patients had UD on the right. Often patients had infections in the urinary tract. Some authors observed hindrance to urine drainage in UD patients. UD symptomatology is almost absent which is confirmed by long-term observations (up to 8–15 years) in four patients with UD. This is explained by the fact that only a few histologic observations are available and no surgeries for UD were carried out. However, two patients had the ureter with UD removed due to other diseases (1, cancer; 1, pyelonephritis). The first observation includes a moderate ureter myopachynsis, and the second observation includes a pseudogonorreha. Prosection of the first patient with UD revealed a minimal external bulging of the ureter wall (Fig. 2.3).

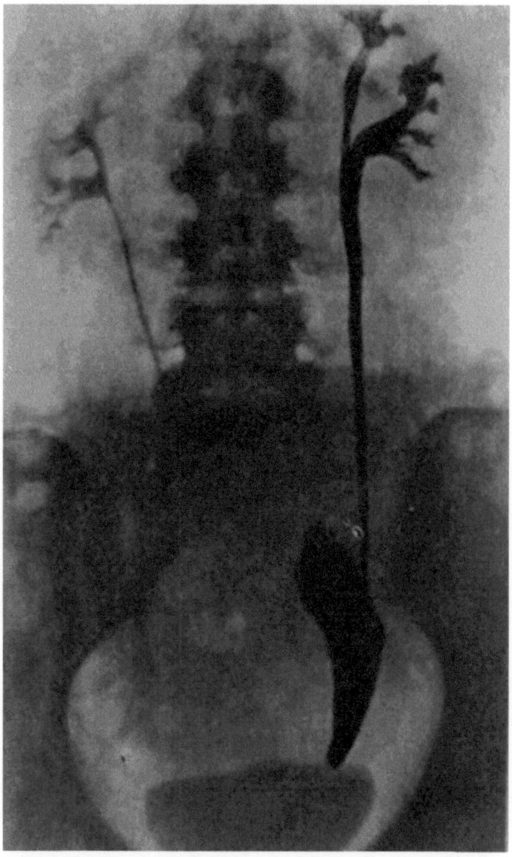

Fig. 2.3 Excretory urogram. Left ureter diverticulum (After Lopatkin and Lyulko [39], Fig. 131, p. 176)

The development of the secondary diverticulum in the part of the left ureter located at the renal pelvis with its congenital valves along with hydronephrosis was described by Kim et al. (2004) (Fig. 2.4).

Ureteral pseudodiverticula can be considered a special type of ureteral diverticula (Fig. 2.5) or periglandular ureteritis (the term used by several authors) [42]. Ureteral pseudodiverticula (UPD) are most often found in men above 50 years old [43–48]. The actual UPD rate is not known. This is attributed to the impossibility to see UPD during EU. Hematuria is the most frequent manifestation which is followed by urological examination. The examination reveals diverticula and in most cases a concurrent infection and/or obstruction of the urinary tract.

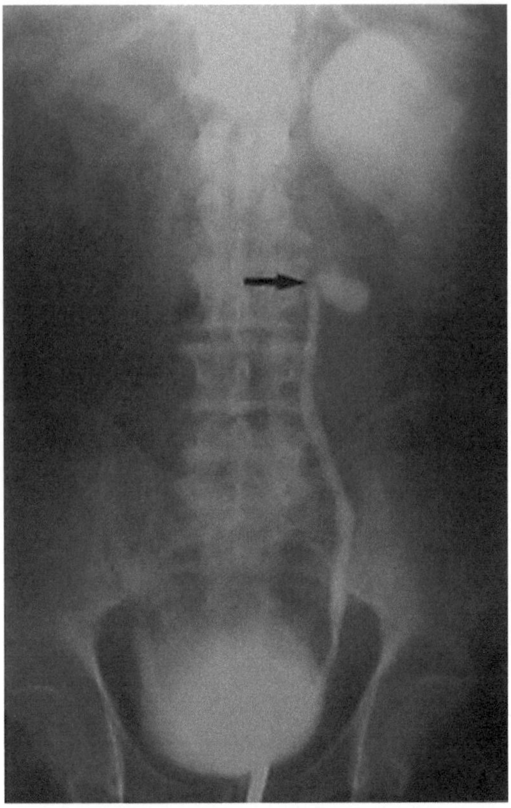

Fig. 2.4 Retrograde ureteropyelogram in case of congenital obstruction of the ureter caused by ureteral valves in a 66-year-old male, namely, compression and constriction of the proximal part of the left ureter caused by valves (shown by the *arrow*) with a prominent hydronephrosis and formation of a diverticulum in the proximal part of the left ureter (After Kim et al. [52])

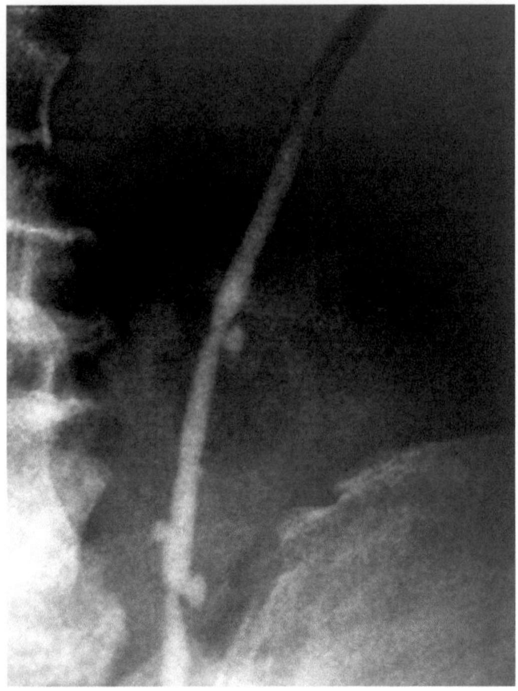

Fig. 2.5 Pseudodiverticula of the left ureter in a retrograde ureterogram in case of ureteral valves (After Kim et al. [52])

As was mentioned above, UD are traditionally divided into two categories: congenital and acquired UD. Congenital (true) diverticula are usually solitary and contain all layers of the normal ureter wall, while the walls of acquired (false) UD consist only of the muscle layer. Histologic examination of multiple UPD reveals that these diverticula do not fall within any of the categories since such "outpouchings" do not consist of the complete ureter wall nor do they prolapse through the muscle layer. Since there is no certainty whether UPD are congenital or acquired, they are probably a metaplastic or hyperplastic reaction of the transitional epithelium which appears due to inflammation and may be part of cystic pyeloureteritis presentation. Actually, the combination of acquired diverticula with a stricture or defect of urinoexcretory system filling more likely means presence of a tumor.

X-ray diagnosis should imply differentiation with the filling defect, imprint, or other disorders caused by cystic ureteritis, tuberculous ureteritis, schistosomatosis, multiple polyposes, atresia, or an external compression of the ureter by varicosity or an accessory artery. Tuberculosis may cause a combination of defects and diverticulum-like changes as well as strictures. Cystic ureteritis usually affects the renal pelvis, while tuberculosis affects both the renal pelvis and calyces. A secondary neoplasm in the ureter may also produce presentation of a small nonmalignant UPD.

Although UPD alone do not require treatment, they may be clinically related to stones, obstruction, infections, and malignant changes of the uroepithelium. It is advisable to monitor UPD by means of cystoscopy performed every year or 6 months and possible cytological examinations of the ureter (Figs. 2.6 and 2.7).

Ureteral pseudodiverticuloses (*UPD*) after Wasserma [48] are cavities up to 5 mm in diameter

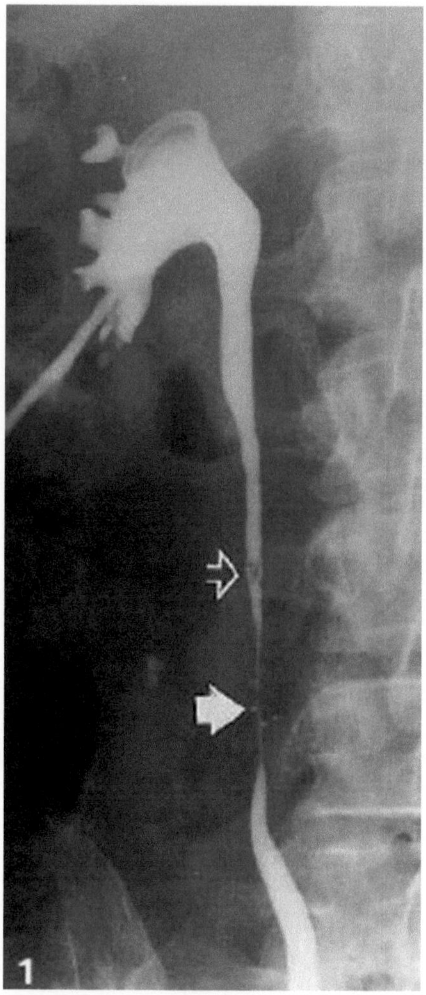

Fig. 2.6 Antegrade pyeloureterogram made by means of a nephrostomic drainage in a 77-year-old patient with pains in the right side and microhematuria in anamnesis displays a minor defect of ureter filling due to a concrement (*open arrow*). Several UPD are present to the distal side form the concrement (*closed arrow*). Recovery after remote lithotripsy (After Department of Radiology, ST George's Hospital, London [42])

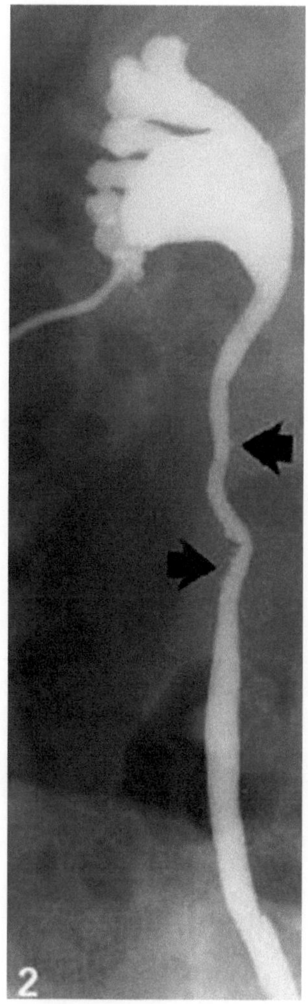

Fig. 2.7 Antegrade ureterogram in a 74-year-old patient with three episodes of hematuria for the last months—stasis of the contrast medium in the right ureter caused by obstruction of the vesicoureteral anastomosis and multiple UPD in the proximal third of the ureter (*arrows*). Cystoscopy did not reveal urinary bladder tumor. Needle biopsy of the prostate gland revealed prostate cancer (After Department of Radiology, ST George's Hospital, London [42])

filled with liquid and connected with the ureter duct. They can be singular, multiple, and uni- and/or bilateral. Usually they are discovered "accidentally" during contrast examination of the urinary tract for benign prostatic hyperplasia, hematuria, renal colic, infections, and urinary tract tumors. In 25 % of ureteral pseudodiverticula (UPD) cases, pseudodiverticula are reported to develop synchronously or metachronously with urothelial cancer. The most frequent type of this cancer is the transitional cell carcinoma, which is localized in the urinary bladder. However, the transitional cell carcinoma can be found both in the ureter and in the renal pelvis and calyces, while the squamous type of the urothelial carcinoma may be associated with UPD.

Very small UD can be found in 11 % of obtained pathologicoanatomic ureter samples where they can be seen thorough visual examination as small dots. As proved by microscopic examinations, small UPD are formed due to ectasia of the hyperplastic submucosal Brunn glands which are directly connected with the ureter

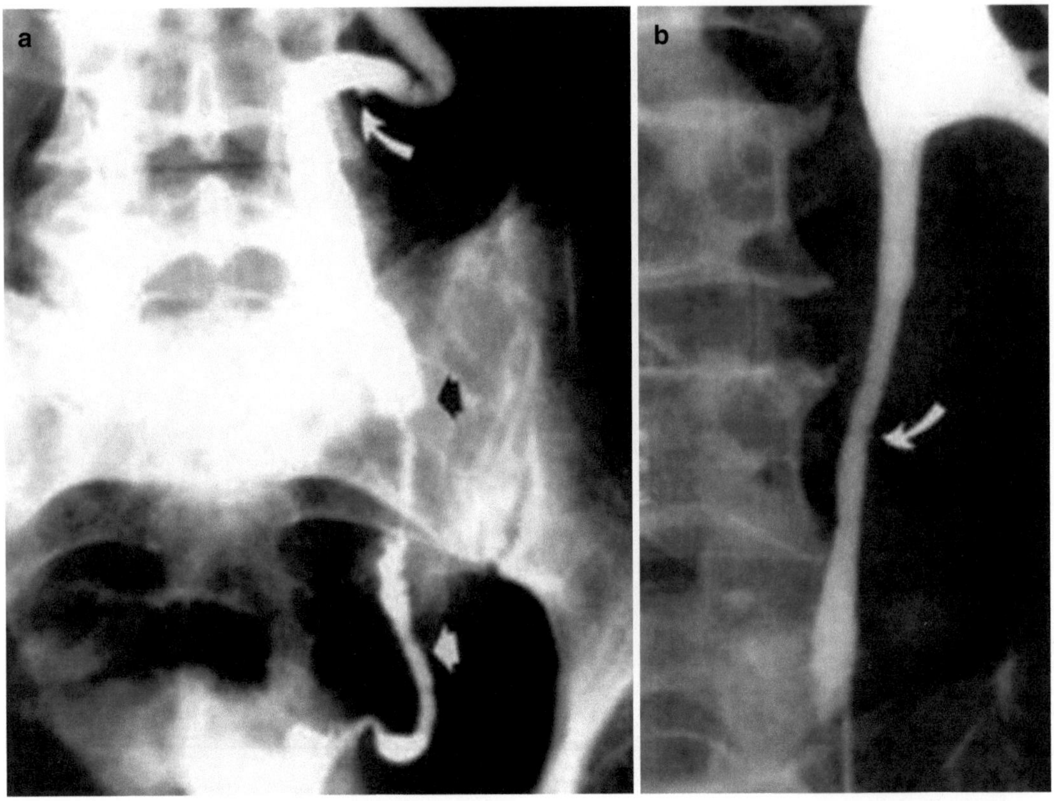

Fig. 2.8 (**a**, **b**) Retrograde ureterograms, left side, of a 73-year-old male the next day after a hematuria episode; a singular UPD is visible (*bent arrows*) combined with squamous cell carcinoma of the distal part of the ureter (between the *short arrows*). Later development of urothelial carcinoma in the urinary bladder discovered (After Wasserman et al. [46])

lumen. Moreover, in the areas affected by UPD formation, microscopic examinations reveal signs of cystic ureteritis which are combined with changes of the abovementioned glands. This fact confirms the statement that UPD result from chronic inflammation. Also the number of discovered UPD increases along with the development of obstruction in the lower part of the urinary tract or along with the development of chronic reflux that causes increased pressure in the ureter lumen.

UPD are best seen in retrograde urograms, but they may also be discovered during intravenous urography. Recently they started to visualize and diagnose UD during multidetector SCTU.

It must be noted that not only correct diagnostics of UPD is of importance, but the doctor or urologist must also be aware of significance of comprehensive patient examination in order to exclude urothelial cancer, including cystoscopy and cytological urine analysis for atypical cells. The second important aspect is that negative data may come from uncertain results of examination in case of metachronous development of urothelial cancer in the ureter and/or the urinary bladder which may develop more than 10 years after UPD discovery.

Combination of UPD with urothelial malignization is possible in approximately 50 % of cases. The presence of UPD in patients with a radiotransparent defect of urinary tract filling indicates a possible malignant transformation in about 71 % of UPD cases. The latter is a representative clinical marker of the upcoming development of a urothelial carcinoma with its further development within 2–10 years. Malignant transformations usually represent urothelial carcinoma of the urinary bladder; however, the first reported cases of UPD were associated with squamous cell carcinoma (Fig. 2.8). There is no correlation between the number of UPD discovered and the possibility of its association with malignization (Figs. 2.8, 2.9, and 2.10).

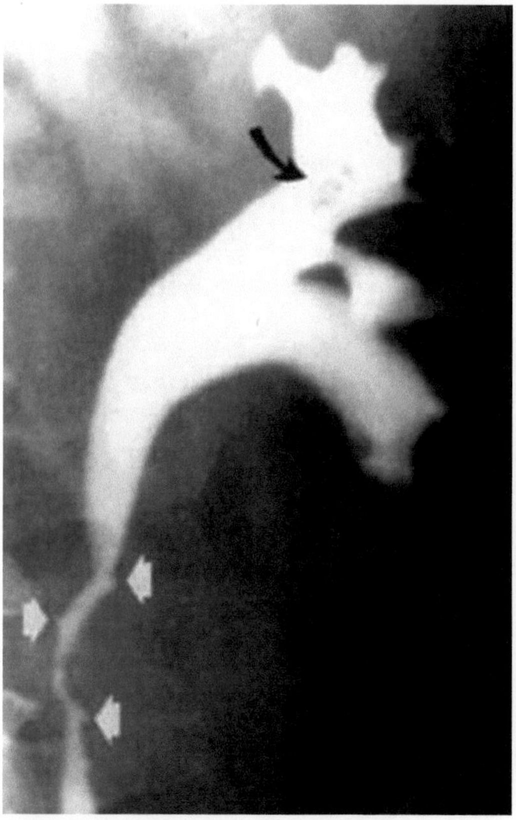

Fig. 2.9 Retrograde ureterogram, left side, of a 74-year-old male with hematuria; a ureteral pseudodiverticulum is seen (*white arrows*) combined with a defect of filling of an upper calyx on the left (*black arrow*). A histologic examination of a surgical sample revealed presence of urothelial cancer (After Wasserman et al. [46])

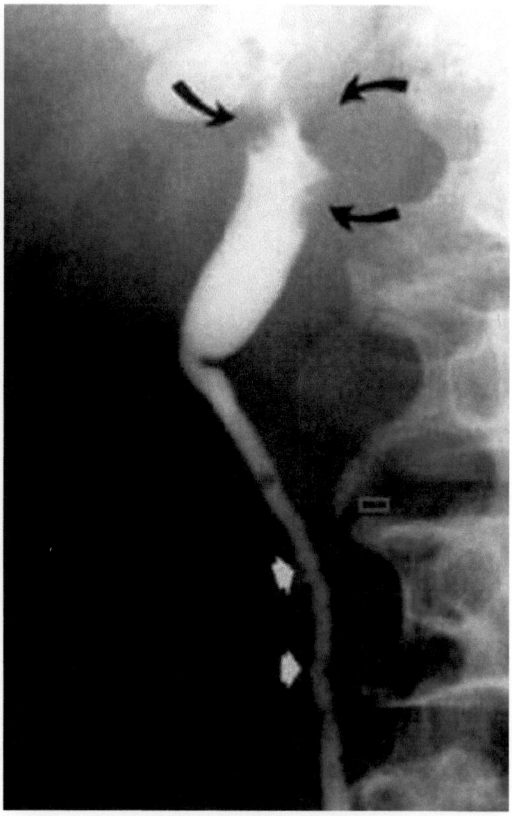

Fig. 2.10 Retrograde ureterogram, right side, of a 63-year-old male with hematuria shows a combination of UPD with a defect of pelvis filling on the right (*black arrows*) caused by obstructive caliectasis. A histologic examination of a surgical sample revealed presence of a stricture and urothelial carcinoma (After Wasserman et al. [46])

Therefore, a convincingly documented presence of UPD may serve as a serious symptom of a potential synchronous or metachronous development of a tumor [45–48].

In our experience we saw a patient who had been diagnosed with a diverticulum in the lower third of the ureter based on EU results; however, that diagnosis was not confirmed by the further examination (Figs. 2.11, 2.12, 2.13, and 2.14).

2.1 Description of the Observation

A 45-year-old woman was admitted to the urological clinic of the Yaroslavl Medical Academy on June 30, 2007, with complaints of pain in the left lumbar area, nausea, and vomiting. The symptoms appeared 3 h earlier. The patient was delivered to the clinic by an ambulance team with the directional diagnosis of the left-side renal colic. A similar presentation was observed in the anamnesis 10 years ago when during examination and treatment in the urological clinic, the patient was diagnosed with urolithiasis. Physical examination displayed a satisfactory general condition of the patient. The abdomen was soft, and palpation revealed pain in the area of the left kidney. Pulse was 76 heartbeats per minute, and arterial blood pressure—130/80 mmHg. Otherwise no abnormal changes of internal organs were discovered. Clinical blood analysis is normal. Clinical urine analysis shows the following results: straw color; specific gravity, 1005; reaction, acid; transparency, presence of

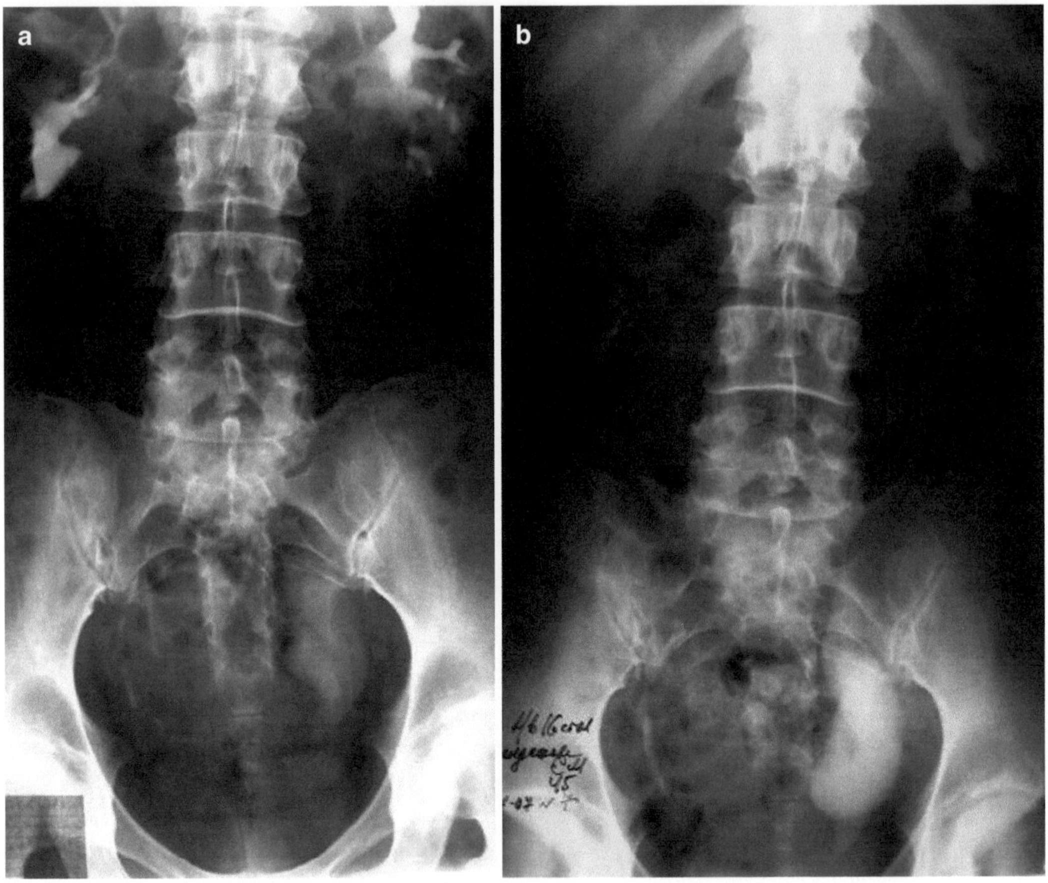

Fig. 2.11 (**a**, **b**) Excretory urograms in the 15th and 16th min (in the vertical position), incomplete rotation of the right kidney and ectasia of the lower part of the left ureter which was interpreted as a diverticulum

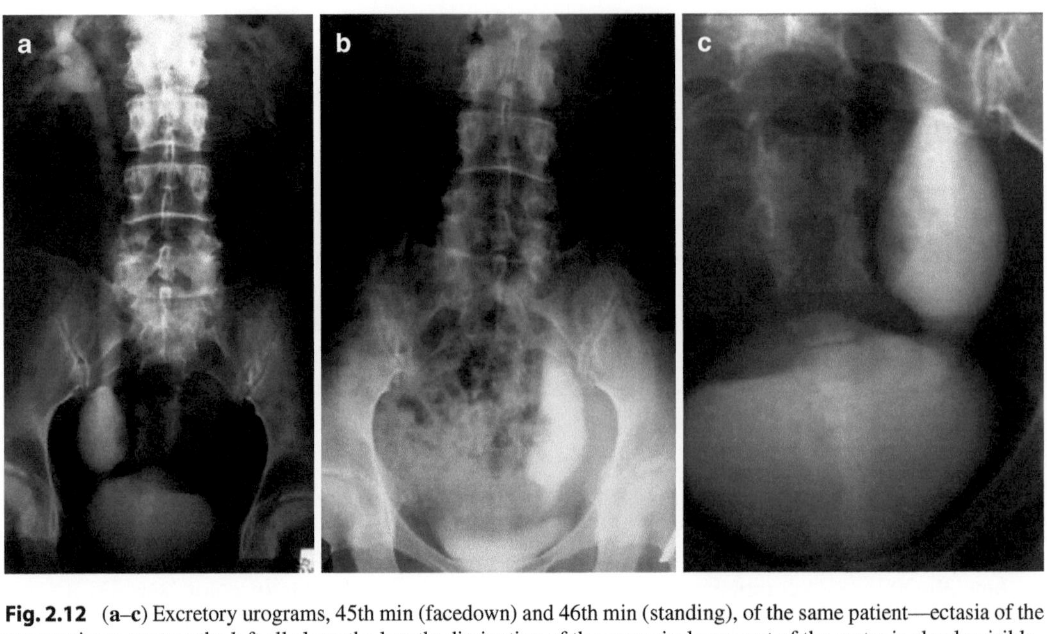

Fig. 2.12 (**a**–**c**) Excretory urograms, 45th min (facedown) and 46th min (standing), of the same patient—ectasia of the upper urinary tract on the left all along the length; diminution of the prevesical segment of the ureter is clearly visible

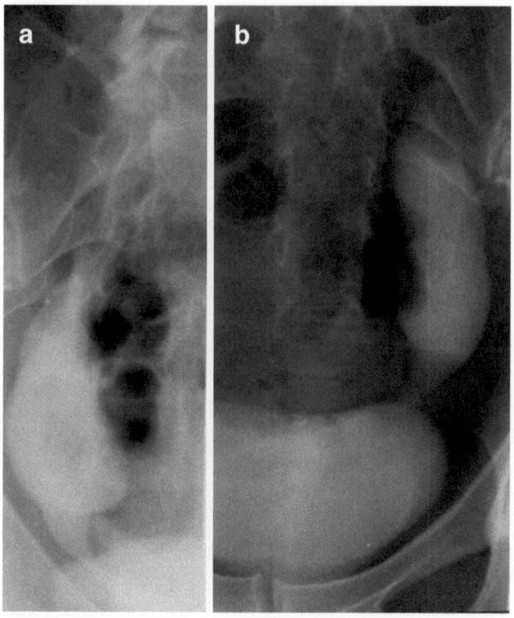

Fig. 2.13 (**a**, **b**) Target ureterograms of the left ureter made under cineradiographic monitoring, the 60th min (facedown) and the 61st min (faceup), of the same patient—ectasia in the prevesical segment of the ureter changes its shape at multiple-view cineradiographic examination, under conditions of functional Valsalva and Muller tests; the distal segment of the ureter narrows in the shape of a "pen" or "mouse tail"

complete, epithelial cells (squamous—in a big amount); multiform cells, 2–3 in sight; leukocytes, 0–1 in sight; and erythrocytes, 2–3 in sight. In the plain film of the urinary tract, a shadow 0.2×0.3 cm similar to a concrement could be seen in the projection of the lower third of the left ureter. Results of ultrasound examination shows the following: for the left side, the kidney is 11.2×6.7 cm in diameter; has hypoechoic parenchyma, 2.0–2.2 cm width, and lobular structure, and is "edematic." The pelvicalyceal system is ectatic, and renal pelvis 2.4 cm wide, having intrarenal location.

The left ureter up to 0.7 cm wide is visible due to prominent meteorism up to the iliac vessels. For the right side, the kidney is 10.7×4.7 cm in diameter and has a normal location, hypoechoic parenchyma, and normal width. No ectasia of pelvicalyceal system is present: size 1.4–1.6 cm. In the middle segment an incomplete parenchyma tectum was discovered. No changes in the urinary bladder were present. The conclusions are ureteropyelocaliectasis on the left side and left-side pyelonephritis. In excretory urograms in the 10th, 16th (standing), and 45th min (Fig. 2.1a, b), the kidneys are located in the normal area and not enlarged. The pelvicalyceal systems are opacified on both sides and not ectatic. After an orthostatic test, a sizeable saccular formation with a sharp outline was opacified in the distal part of the ectatic left ureter. The ureter and pelvicalyceal systems remain ectatic in the vertical position. The conclusions are ureteropyelocaliectasis and a large ureteral diverticulum on the left. The follow-up ultrasound examination performed after antispasmodic and anti-inflammatory therapy revealed a decrease in the width of the left kidney parenchyma down to 1.8 cm; no signs of the parenchymal edema were discovered. No ectasia of the pelvicalyceal system is present.

In order to clarify the condition of the left ureter, a repeated examination was carried out, namely, excretory urography with cineradiographic ureteropyeloscopy (Fig. 2.8a–c): In excretory urograms, the 25th min (faceup, facedown, and in the vertical position), as well as in multiple-view cineradiograms in the 45th min, under conditions of Valsalva and Muller tests and after urination *on the right*, the kidney is moderately rotated anteriorly and to the medial side (calyceal fornices are partly orientated anteriorly and medially; the pelvicalyceal system is located laterally). In the vertical position, the kidney descends more than two vertebral bodies. The orthostatic reaction of the upper urinary tract is of the eutonic type. Normal location, shape, and size are on the left side. The upper urinary tract is ectatic all along its length; some parts of calyceal fornices are smoothed and rounded. The greatest (up to 3.5 cm) ectasia of the ureter is observed in its lower third which forms an additional loop that is the most intensively opacified when the patient is lying facedown and standing. Under conditions of tests implying increase of the abdominal pressure and after urination, a deep peristalsis in the pelvic part of the ureter is observed, sometimes with regurgitation of the contrast medium into the upper third of the ureter and into the renal pelvis. The intravesical part of the ureter has the appearance of a

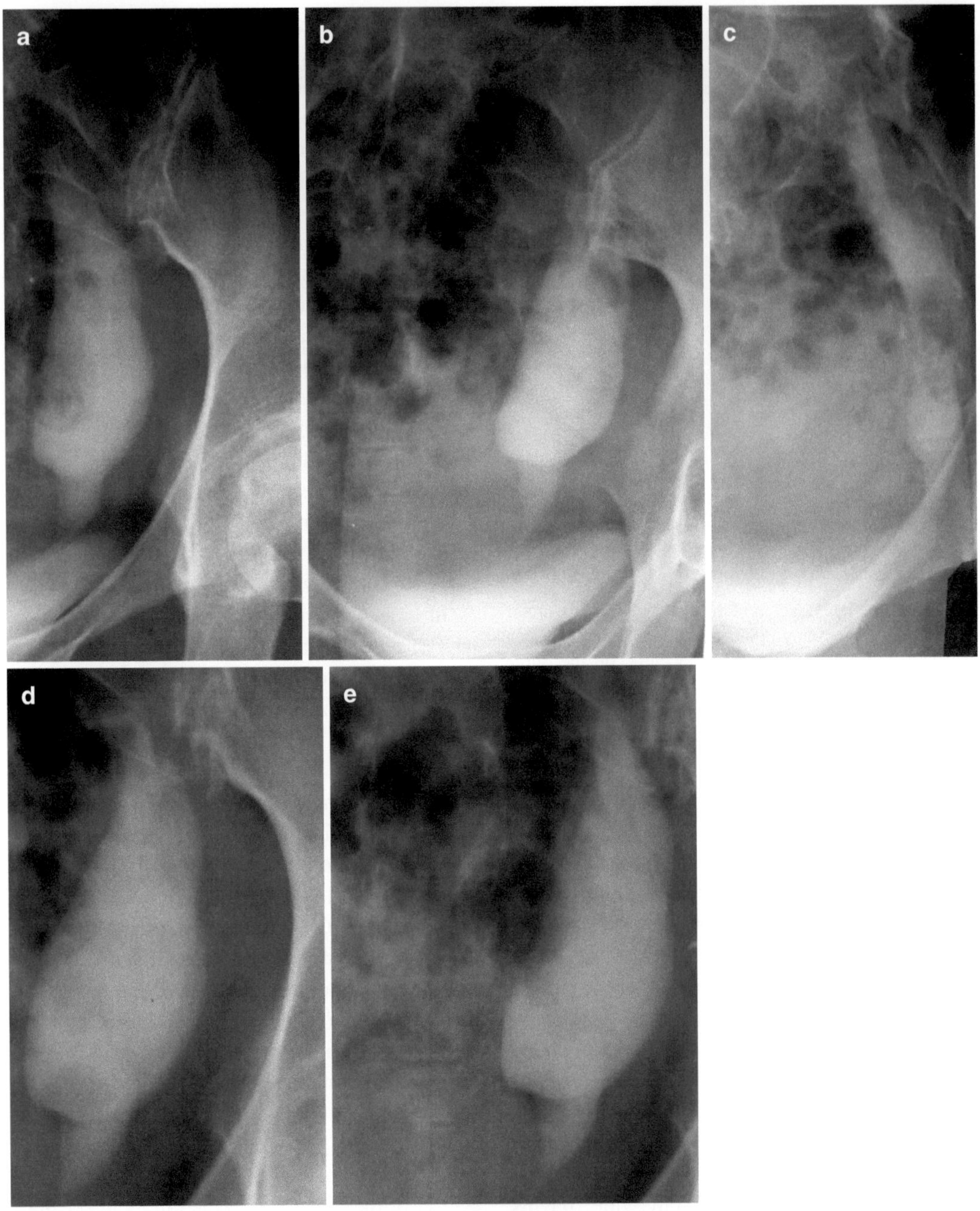

Fig. 2.14 (**a**–**e**) Target ureterograms made under cineradiographic monitoring, the 60th min (*vertical position*) after an intravenous contrast medium injection, of the same patient—ectasia of the prevesical segment of the ureter in the form of an additional loop changes its shape at multiple-view cineradiographic examination, under conditions of functional Valsalva and Muller tests; vesical segment of the ureter narrows in the shape of a "pen" or "mouse tail"

"mouse tail." The urinary bladder in the descending cystogram is unchanged. The conclusions are a bilateral abnormality of kidneys and of the upper urinary tract in the form of incomplete rotation and nephroptosis on the right without disturbance of urodynamics. Achalasia of the intravesical part of

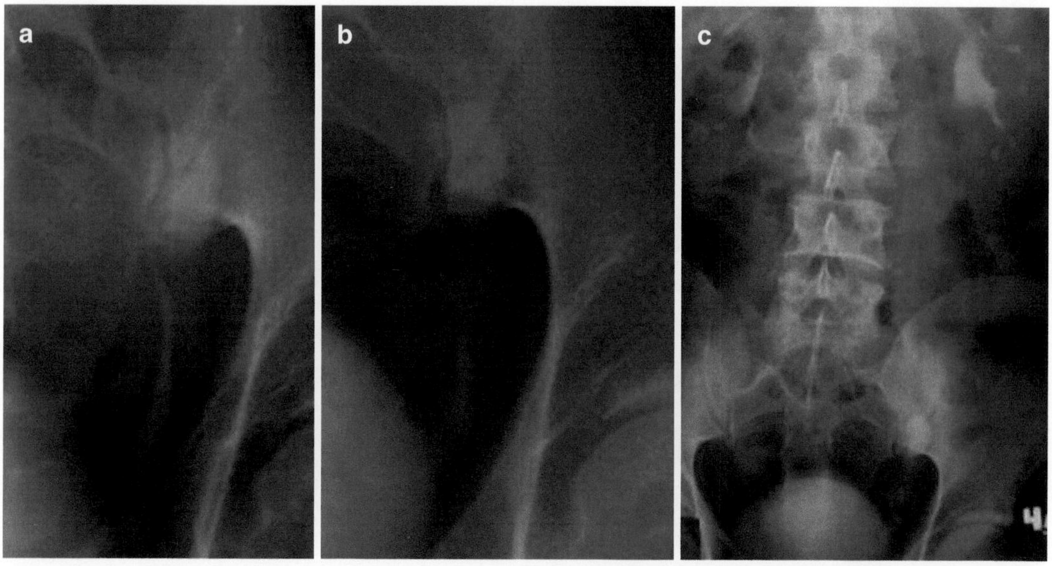

Fig. 2.15 (**a**) Excretory urogram, 45th min; (**b**, **c**) target excretory urograms under cineradiographic monitoring, 60th min—(**b**) in the vertical position, (**c**) in the horizontal position faceup

the left ureter is complicated with a prominent ureteropyelectasis with an additional loop in the lower third of the ureter, vesicoureteral reflux, and signs of chronic left-side pyelonephritis.

For more than 30 years of work in urological clinics, we observed only one patient with a congenital UD in the lower third of the left ureter [49–51].

The 47-year-old man was admitted to the urological clinic for verification of his diagnosis and so that a decision concerning his occupational fitness can be made (the patient worked as a carman). Preventive abdominal and retroperitoneum ultrasound, which was the first in the patient's life, revealed small concrements (up to 0.3–0.5 cm) in the pelvicalyceal structure of both kidneys and a moderate pyelocaliectasis on the left. The patient did not have any complaints. Clinical and laboratory data were within the norm.

A congenital UD in the prevesical part of the left ureter was diagnosed by means of excretory urography combined with dynamic IVU with fluoroscopy. During the examination an additional ovoid 1.5×2.0 cm cavity with sharp outlines was discovered which was connected with the lateral wall of the prevesical part of the left ureter and had a weak wall peristalsis which could be observed along with contractions of the ureter cystoids (Fig. 2.15). During plain CAT examination of the kidneys and prevesical part of the ureter, concrements varying from 0.3 to 0.5 cm were discovered in both kidneys, and also an additional round formation was revealed in the projection of the prevesical part of the left ureter which was 1.0 in diameter and contained a concrement 0.2 cm in diameter (Fig. 2.16).

In T2-weighted MRI in the coronal projection, also spina bifida of vertebral body L-4 and a moderate left-side pyelectasis were discovered (Fig. 2.17).

Plain MRI/MRU carried out by means of a low-field MR imaging unit (Signa Profile HD 0.2 T Open MRI System, GE Healthcare) revealed a similar presentation with UD increased after the introduction of Lasix. MRU in the coronal and especially in the sagittal projection, along with a typical presentation of UD in the lower third of the left ureter, revealed a small Tarlov cyst. Such a cyst is a kind of sacral meningocele; it has a form of extradural cyst of perineural localization which is not connected with the arachnoid cavity and results from a diverticulum of the pachymeninx (Fig. 2.18).

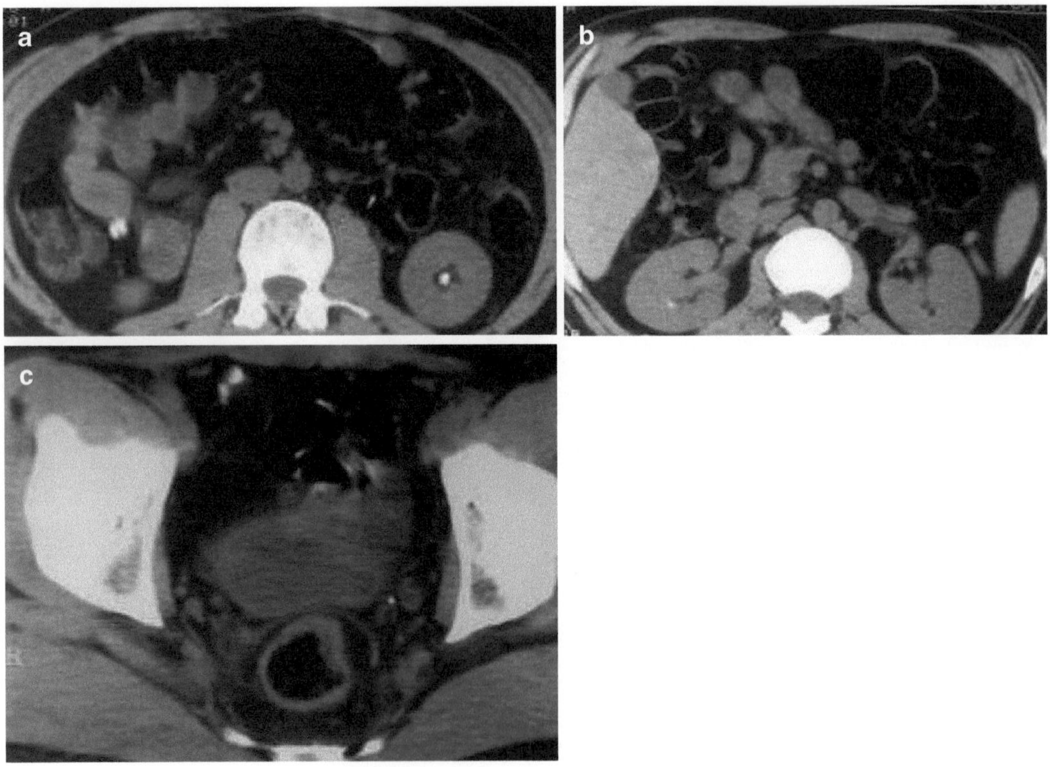

Fig. 2.16 (**a**–**c**) CT images: (**a**) stones in the lower calyx of the left kidney diameter about 0.5 and 0.2 cm; (**b**) a stone in a middle calyx of the right kidney, diameter about 0.3 cm; (**c**) a stone in a projection of diverticulum in the lower third of the left ureter

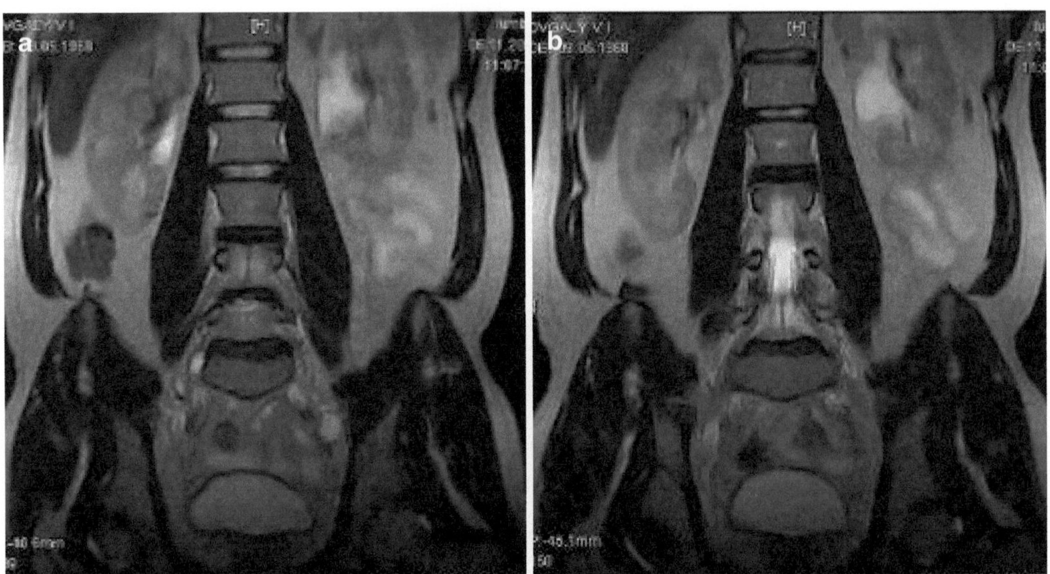

Fig. 2.17 (**a**, **b**) T2-weighted MRI in the coronal projection—(**a**) spina bifida of vertebral body L-4; (**b**) moderate left-side pyelectasis

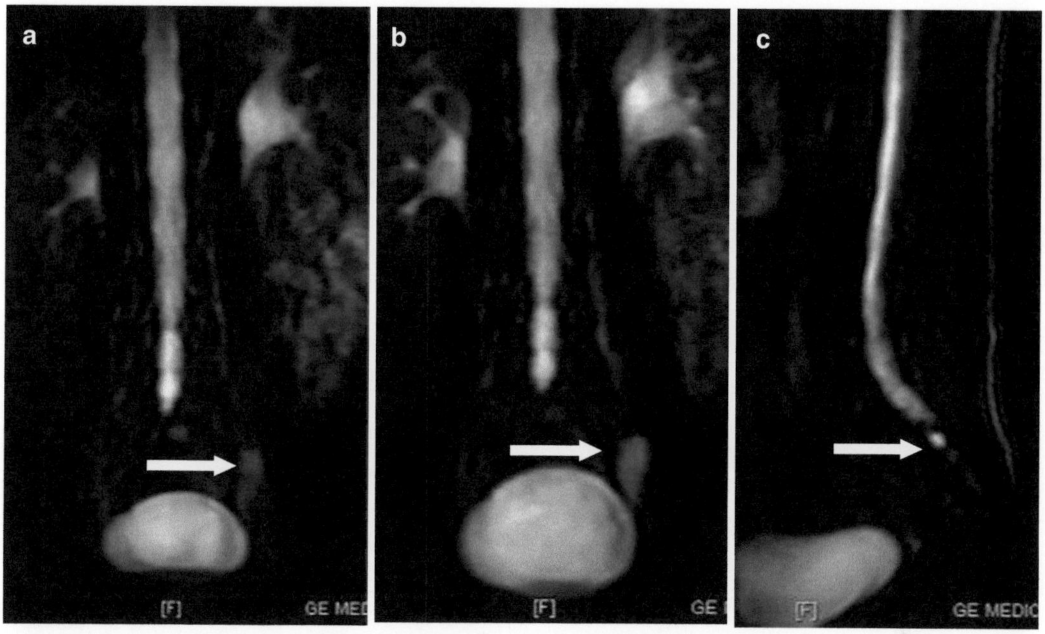

Fig. 2.18 (**a**, **b**) MRU in the coronal projection before and after intravenous injection of Lasix, an additional ovoid shadow in the projection of the prevesical part of the left ureter which expanded after Lasix injection (*arrows*); (**c**) MRU in the sagittal projection, Tarlov cyst (*arrow*)

The presence of UD was confirmed by means of a repeated target USG with colored Doppler mapping and a 3D image reconstruction on EnVisor ultrasound scanner (Philips, Germany) after furosemide intake. An additional 1.0×2.0 cm ovoid formation was detected which was located near the prevesical part of the ureter. It filled in 25 min after furosemide intake and emptied together with the urinary bladder (Fig. 2.19).

All that confirmed the congenital nature of the changes discovered. The proposal to do retrograde urography of the left side in order to confirm UD diagnosis was considered impractical due to enough credibility of the results obtained by noninvasive ray diagnostics. Moreover, the application of an invasive instrumental method of examination, which is retrograde urography, was contradicted due to the fact that the patient was getting treatment with anticoagulants for thrombophlebitis of deep veins of the lower limbs. The patient was discharged from the hospital under the supervision of the dispensary urologist.

Our observation shows a high informational value of EU that reveals UD as a globular or saccular additional cavity with sharp outlines directly adjoining the ureter which is constricted in that area. Rate of the contrast medium accumulation in the UD cavity increases in delayed images, and UD opacification is preserved even after discharge of the contrast medium from the upper urinary tract.

The observation described above for the first time also demonstrates high diagnostic efficiency of plain MRU performed by means of a low-field tomography with a preliminary intravenous Lasix injection. A no less efficient method was a repeated target USG in a urological clinic with a preliminary intake of furosemide which was carried out by a doctor upon studying the results of the preceding IVU and MRU.

In majority of patients, clinical presentations appear as late as above 20 years old and are as follows: pains, overlay of urinary tract infections, lithogenesis, and, in very rare cases, development of tumors in the UD cavity [32] or simulation of tumors by large UD in the pelvic cavity [33, 36].

Congenital UD, the same as in the described observation, can be combined with spine and spinal cord abnormalities [34, 35].

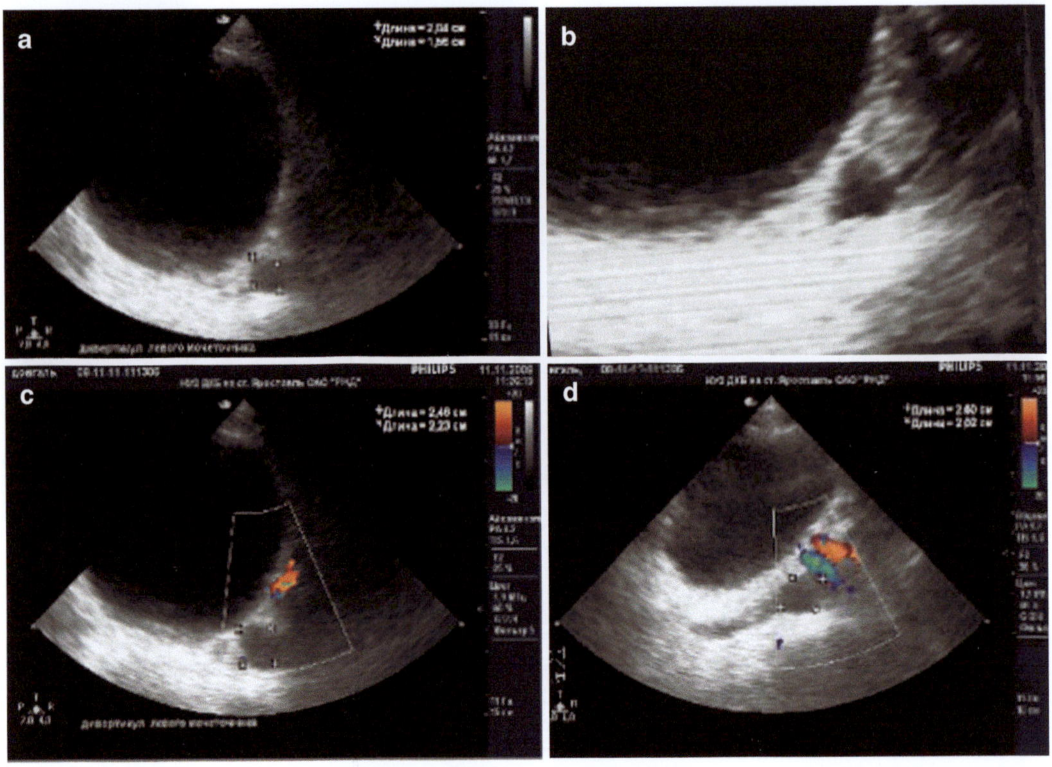

Fig. 2.19 (**a–d**) Sonograms: (**a**) in the grayscale mode; (**b**) in 3D mode; (**c, d**) in the colored Doppler mapping mode: a diverticulum of the prevesical part of the left ureter. In the small pelvis to the lateral side from the urinary bladder, in the projection of the prevesical part of the ureter, on the left, an additional anechogenic oval formation, 1.5 × 2.2 × 2.5 cm, is seen. The formation has sharp outlines and smooth boundaries and produces a weak effect of dorsal increase of the echo signal; it has a homogenous structure and looks nonvascular in the colored Doppler mapping mode

Treatment of UD consists of conservative therapy for inflammatory infections which may develop in the diverticulum cavity due to its hindered drainage. Surgical treatment is used only in case of severe pain syndrome, obstinate pyuria, and disturbed urodynamics in the urinary tract. Diverticulectomy and resection of the perivesical part of the ureter with ureterocystoneoanastomosis are justified only in rare cases, such as giant UD, lithogenesis, and prominent disturbances of urodynamics on the UD side [38–40].

2.2 Algorithm of UD Diagnostics

In our opinion, excretory urography retains the leading position in X-ray imaging, including combination of that method with cineradiography (or dynamic IVU with fluoroscopy), which provides the most detailed information on the anatomical and functional condition of the upper urinary tract all along its length by means of the most accurate and direct analogue imaging.

Our experience confirms that a negative USG result in respect to UD diagnostics does not preclude from performing EU, SCTU, and MRU as the next steps as these are also efficient methods for clarifying the anatomical condition of the UUT. However, these methods do not provide information on the motor function of the upper urinary tract and have a limited availability due to their high cost.

Conclusion

Therefore, as follows from the analysis of the published UD cases and our observations, nowadays, it is possible to diagnose such a rare abnormality as UD by means of the following noninvasive X-ray imaging: EU, especially in the form of dynamic IVU with fluoroscopy; SCT/SCTU; as well as USG and MRI/MRU, including low-field MR imagers, along with the usage of diuretics and without invasive technologies (retrograde ureterography and/or ureteroscopy).

References

1. Culp OS. Ureteral diverticulum: classification of literature and report of an authentic case. J Urol. 1947; 58:309.
2. Chen M-H, Lee Y-H, Huang J-K. Ureteral pseudodiverticulosis: report of two cases. J Urol ROC. 2000;11: 67–70.
3. McGraw AB, Culp OS. Diverticulum of the ureter: report of another authentic case. J Urol. 1952;67:262.
4. Harlin H, Atkinson H. Ureteral diverticulum. Urol Cutan Rev. 1950;54(9):526–31.
5. Desgrez JP. Diverticulose ureterale. Ann Urol. 1983;17(2):96–8.
6. Tokunaka S, Koyanagi T, Matusuna T, et al. Paraureteral diverticula: clinical experience with 17 cases with associated renal dysmorphism. J Urol. 1980;124(6):791–6.
7. Davidov MI, Lyadov AA, Lyadov SA. Ureteral abnormalities Lib.: plenary session of the Board of the Russian Society of Urologists. Materials, St. Petersburg, 29–31 Oct 2008. p. 239–40.
8. Yoshida S, Nakagomi K, Goto S. A case of true ureteral diverticulum [article in Japanese]. Nippon Hinyokika Gakkai Zasshi. 2005;96(1):25–8.
9. Sklifosovsky NV. Demonstration of a hydronephrosis preparation with a ureteral diverticulum. Chronicles Surg Soc Moscow. 1887;7(2–3):c. 22–3.
10. Delmas J, Delmas P. Sur les anomalies ureterales. Ann Maland Org genitor-urin. 1910;28:9–15.
11. Gotlib YG. Ureteral diverticula. Urology. 1927;4(2): 45–50.
12. Ovchinnikov NM. A case of a stone in a ureteral diverticulum. Urology. 1927;4(3):46–8.
13. Tshvetadze YO, Fainstein DD. Revisited ureteral diverticulum. Soviet Surg. 1934;7(4):216–9.
14. Tshvetadze YO. Two cases of ureteral diverticulum. Urology. 1936;13(2):216–9.
15. Richardson EH. Diverticulum of the ureter: a collective review with report of an unique example. J Urol. 1942;47:535–6.
16. Rank WB, Mellinger GT, Spiro E. Ureteral diverticula: etiologic considerations. J Urol. 1960;83:566–8.
17. Zhukov MN, Klyucharyov BV, Rozhdestvensky V. Lib.: surgical disorders of kidneys and ureters, Leningrad: Meditsina; 1965. p. 91–2.
18. Baldanov S. Ureteral diverticulum. Materials of reports of Science and Practice Conference of Doctors of the Zabaikalsk Railway (June 25–26, 1970), P. 1. Chita; 1970. p. 122–5.
19. Rzheznikov MS. Congenital ureteral diverticulum. Urol Nephrol. 1974;(1):38–41.
20. Larrett D, Malek R. Ureteral diverticulum. J Urol. 1975;114:33–5.
21. Ostropolskaya EA, Osipov IB, Akhmedshin I. Ureteral diverticulum. Urol Nephrol. 1977;(2):65–6.
22. Franco I, Choudhury M, Eshghi M, Bhalodi A, Addonizio JC. Fibroepithelial polyp associated with congenital ureteral diverticulum: report of 2 cases. J Urol. 1988;140:598–600.
23. Cope RM, Snow BW. Massive cystic ureteral diverticula in infancy. J Urol. 1991;146:575–7.
24. Greed L, Post J, Hillman B, et al. Multiple ureteral diverticula. Urol Radiol. 1980;2(1):29–32.
25. Savchenko NE, Sklabeyus IA. Ureteral diverticula. Lib.: conference of urologists of Lith. SSR. 2nd ed. Materials of reports. Kaunas; 1977. p. 206–8.
26. Marcos FH, Rocha J, Marconi T, et al. Congenital ureteral diverticulum. Int Braz J Urol. 2000;26(4): 403–5.
27. Holly LE, Sumcad B. Diverticular ureteral changes: a report of 4 cases. AJR Am J Roentgenol. 1957;78: 1053–60.
28. Aivazyan AV, Vojno-Yasenetsky AM. Development abnormalities of kidneys and ureters. M. Nauka. 1988. Subtype B. Ureteral diverticulum. p. 329–33.
29. Johnin K. Congenital ureteral diverticulum coexistent with hydronephrosis caused by vascular compression involving the uterine artery and umbilical ligament: report of a case. J Pediatr Surg. 2003;35(9):1350–2.
30. Kumar S. Multiple ureteral diverticula. J Natl Med Assoc. 1974;66:161–2.
31. Cussenot O, Desgrandchamps F, Teillac P, et al. Double ureter and congenital diverticulum of the ureter. Surg Radiol Anat. 1991;13:323–6.
32. Harrison GS. Transitional cell carcinoma in congenital ureteral diverticulum. J Urol. 1983;129:1231–2.
33. Haberal A, Kovalak EE, Gokcu M, et al. Diverticulum of the ureter presenting as an adnexal mass in a woman with familial adenomatous polyposis. J Turk German Gynecol Assoc. 2006;7(1):34–8.
34. Rai AS, Taylor TKF, Smith GHH, Cumming RG, Plunkett-Cole M. Congenital abnormalities of the urogenital tract in association with congenital vertebral malformations. J Bone Joint Surg [Br]. 2002; 84-B:891–5.
35. Beals RK, Robbins JR, Rolfe B. Anomalies associated with vertebral malformations. Spine. 1993;18: 1329–32.
36. Hsieh DF, Wu HC. A ureteral diverticulum mimicking pelvic cyst. JTUA. 2002;13(4):157–9.
37. Pytel AY, Tchebanyuk GM. Renal and ureteral abnormalities. Clinical urology manual. Under editorship of Pytel AY, Moscow: Meditsina; 1960. p. 231–90.
38. Pytel AY, Pytel YA. X-ray diagnostics of urological diseases. Moscow: Meditsina; 1961. p. 183.
39. Lopatkin NA, Lyulko AV. Abnormalities of urogenital system. Kiev: Zdorovja; 1987.

40. Lester PD, Kyaw MM. Ureteral diverticulosis. Radiology. 1985;106:77–80.
41. Cohran ST, Walsman J, Barbaric ZL. Radiographic and microscopic findings in multiple ureteral diverticula. Radiology. 1980;137:631–6.
42. Ureteral Pseudodiverticulosis: glandular periureteritis. Department of Radiology, ST George's Hospital, London. http://www.uro.ru/knowledge_base/clinical_cases.
43. Wasserman NF, La Pointe S, Posalaky IP. Ureteral pseudodiverticulosis. Radiology. 1985;155(3):561–6.
44. Kenney PJ, Wasserman NF. Ureteral pseudodiverticulosis associated with carcinoma of renal pelvis. Urol Radiol. 1987;9(3):161–3.
45. Wasserman NF, Posalaky IP, Dykosky R. The pathology of ureteral pseudodiverticulosis. Invest Radiol. 1988;23(8):592–8.
46. Wasserman NF, Zhang G, Posalaky IP, Reddy PK. Ureteral pseudodiverticula: frequent association with uroepithelial malignancy. AJR Am J Roentgenol. 1991;157(1):69–72.
47. Wasserman NF. Pseudodiverticulosis: unusual appearance for metastases to the ureter. Abdom Imaging. 1994;19(4):376–8.
48. Wasserman NF. Other inflammatory conditions of the urinary tract. In: 16th European symposium on urogenital radiology, 10–13 Sept 2009, Athens. p. 61–3.
49. Builov VM, Sencha AN. Ultrasonic, urographic, CAT and MRI/MRU diagnostics of ureteral diverticula Lib.: The Neva Radiological Forum, 6–9 Apr 2009, Publishing House of the St. Petersburg State Medical University, St. Petersburg; 2009. p. 99–101.
50. Builov VM, Sencha AN. US, IVU, CT and MRI findings of congenital ureteral diverticulum P48. In: The 16th European Symposium on Urogenital Radiology (ESUR 2009), Athens, 10–13 Sept 2009. p. 148.
51. Builov VM, Sencha AN. Ureteral diverticulum. Urology. 2010;(2):64–6.
52. Kim SH. Ed. Radiology Illustrated Uroradiology Sanders, 2003, p. 87.

3 Diagnostic Imaging of Urinary Bladder Diverticula

Urinary bladder diverticulum (UBD) is an outpouching of the bladder wall creating an additional cavity which is connected by means of a more or less narrow neck with the urinary bladder cavity. The first UBD description and proposed tactics of its treatment is by Morganini and dates back to 1769 [1].

There are true or congenital UBD and false or acquired UBD. True diverticula are usually singular and false ones are multiple. The congenital diverticulum is connected with the urinary bladder cavity by a narrow duct; its wall consists of the same layers as the urinary bladder wall. Urinary bladder diverticula are located most often in the area of ureteral orifices and bladder sidewalls; in rare cases they appear on the bladder top or around its bottom. Often the congenital diverticulum is larger and has a bigger capacity than the urinary bladder. It must be differentiated from such a rare congenital abnormality as the duplicated urinary bladder [2–5].

Several types of the congenital UBD are defined:

(a) Complete duplication of the urinary bladder (synonym: duplicated urinary bladder)—two urethras present. Each of the two bladders has one ureter and is located in the pelvis. Duplicated urinary bladder is often combined with duplication of the colon and rectovaginal fistulas [6].
(b) Incomplete duplication of the urinary bladder—the two bladders have a common neck and urethra.
(c) Complete sagittal or transverse septum of the urinary bladder (synonym: two-chamber urinary bladder)—duplication of the urinary bladder wall without serous membrane, which divides the bladder into two halves. In this situation, one part is obstructive.

In case of duplicated urinary bladder, the bladder is divided into two parts by a longitudinal septum (Fig. 3.1a, b). Every part of the urinary bladder may be individually connected with its own urethra (the case of duplicated urethra); both halves of the bladder may open into a common urethra or only one-half of the bladder opens into the urethra (Fig. 3.1c, d). Diagnosis may be defined based on cystography. The cystogram shows shadows of the two halves of the urinary bladder separated with a septum which has an oval outline in the area of its top. This shape of the bladder shadow is similar to the heart symbol. A still rarer case of abnormality is the sandglass-shaped bladder: In the cystogram the shadow of one-half of the bladder is located above the other in the craniocaudal direction.

False or acquired UBD develop in patients who have had a long-term disturbance of urine discharge from the bladder which appears as urinary difficulty that is most often observed in patients with benign prostate hyperplasia.

3.1 Epidemiology

Congenital UBD are found rarely; according to results of autopsy of children, the rate is 1:100; they are more often found in boys than in girls and much more often in men than in women. The cause

V.M. Builov, *Imaging of Urinary Tract Diverticula*,
DOI 10.1007/978-3-319-05383-7_3, © Springer International Publishing Switzerland 2014

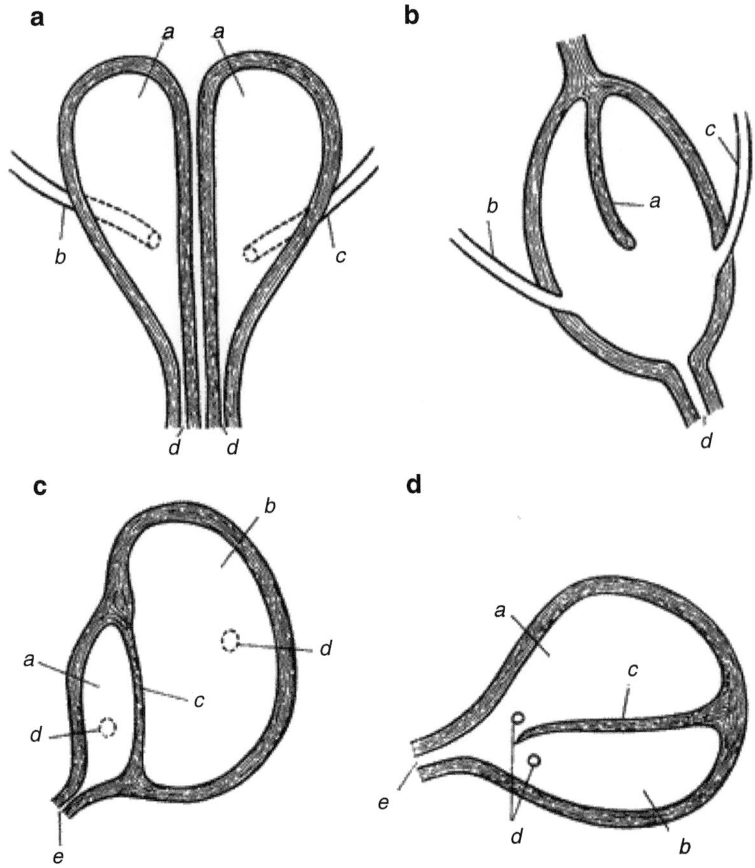

Fig. 3.1 Schemes of complete and incomplete duplication of the urinary bladder. (**a**) Complete duplication of the urinary bladder: *a* urinary bladders, *b* right ureter, *c* left ureter, *d* two individual urethras. (**b**) Incomplete duplication of the urinary bladder: *a* septum, *b* right ureter, *c* left ureter, *d* urethra. (**c**) Complete duplication of the urinary bladder in case a frontal septum is present: *a* front cavity, *b* rear cavity, *c* septum, *d* ureteral orifices, *e* urethra. (**d**) Incomplete duplication of the urinary bladder in case a frontal septum is present: *a* front cavity, *b* rear cavity, *c* septum, *d* ureteral orifices, *e* urethra (After Pytel and Pytel [6])

of congenital UBD formation is supposed to be development abnormality or influence of certain congenital factors such as trauma and retention of urine during the antenatal period. The rate of acquired diverticula development correlates with the incidence of diseases which cause infravesical obstruction (benign prostate hyperplasia, urethra stricture, sclerosis of urinary bladder neck, prostate sclerosis, etc.). It was discovered that every fifth patient which had surgery for infravesical obstruction developed UBD; however, only 15 % of those diverticula required surgical treatment [7–9].

3.2 Classification, Etiology, and Pathogenesis

The most common classification is dividing diverticula into congenital or true diverticula and acquired or false diverticula. The cause of development of true diverticula as the urinary bladder abnormality is malformation of the urinary bladder wall due to the influence of factors such as a trauma and urine retention during the antenatal period. The rate of acquired or false UBD development correlates with the incidence of diseases which cause infravesical obstruction (benign prostate hyperplasia, urethra stricture, sclerosis of urinary bladder neck, prostate sclerosis, etc.). Development of acquired UBD was observed in every fifth patient which had had surgery for infravesical obstruction.

Apart from the etiology of congenital and acquired UBD, the following criteria are also used for their type division: diverticulum wall containing a complete set of layers or only mucosa, number of diverticula and their size, presence or absence of a sphincter, etc. This classification implies different etiologies of true and false diverticula. The former are considered to be a consequence of dysembryogenesis, and the latter—a result of infravesical obstruction. However, there is a number of works where this classification is subject to valid criticism. The provided evidence includes observations of acquired diverticula that contained a full set of layers characteristic of the bladder wall and of congenital diverticula that consisted only of mucosa. In this case the etiology of acquired and congenital diverticula looks similar—formation of diverticula depends on two factors: congenital, weakness of certain parts of the urinary bladder, and acquired, urinary difficulty.

Anatomical features which before were considered as parameters for UBD classification into congenital and acquired ones, such as different structure of walls of congenital and acquired diverticula, presence of a sphincter in the congenital diverticulum neck, and multiplicity of acquired diverticula, are considered to be invalid by the majority of authors, since congenital and acquired UBD cannot be differentiated from each other at the morphological level [10, 11].

A similar study of the urinary bladder wall revealed that the wall was not developed equally in all parts of the bladder [3]. Noted that "...the urinary bladder has parts, where diverticula are found most often (area of ureteral orifices, the front and the rear walls), that feature a weaker development of muscles..." [3]. As for the sphincter of the diverticulum, the majority of authors deem that it is formed by connivent muscles of detrusor; thus, it cannot be called a true sphincter. Contractions of the detrusor during urination prevent the diverticulum from complete voiding, and residual urine accumulates in it. This caused describing UBD as "urine trap." In spite of differences in views on UBD etiology, it should be said that up to now division of diverticula into true and false ones is the most common classification.

Thus, UBD can develop both during antenatal and postnatal life; however, the mechanism of their formation is the same: on the one hand, a weakness of certain bladder parts and, on the other hand, an obstruction to the bladder voiding (Figs. 3.1 and 3.2).

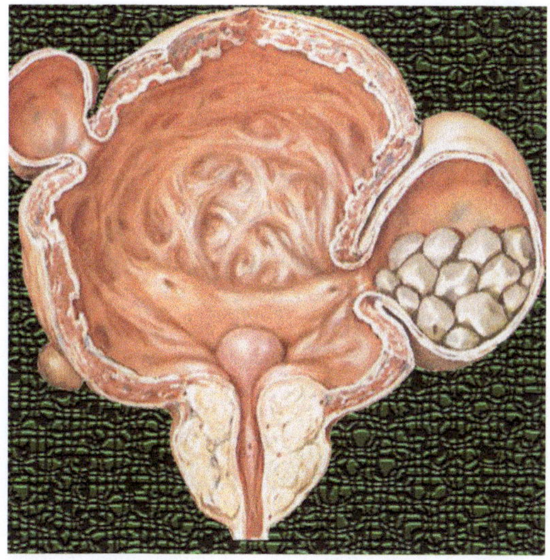

Fig. 3.2 Urinary bladder diverticula resulting from urinary difficulty which was caused by prostate adenoma (trilobe hyperplasia, detrusor hypertrophy). Stones in the diverticulum

3.3 Clinical Diagnostics

In case no symptoms appear, which is typical for the majority of UBD cases, the diverticulum is discovered "accidentally," nowadays most often during USG examinations. Previously UBD were incidentally discovered during cystoscopy or cystography.

Many authors note that in case of UBD no typical clinical presentations are observed and infravesical obstruction symptoms prevail mostly.

The main UBD symptoms are urinary difficulty (up to complete urine retention), two-stage urination (urine is discharged first from the bladder and then from the diverticulum), or urination with Courvoisier procedure; these symptoms are observed not often.

UBD clinical presentations are induced by complications of this disease, such as overlay of infections and lithogenesis, compression of adjacent organs, hematuria, and ureterohydronephrosis. Vesicoureteral reflux may develop if the diverticulum is located in the area of ureteral orifice when its closing function is affected. Until complications arise, the diverticulum usually remains completely latent [5, 10].

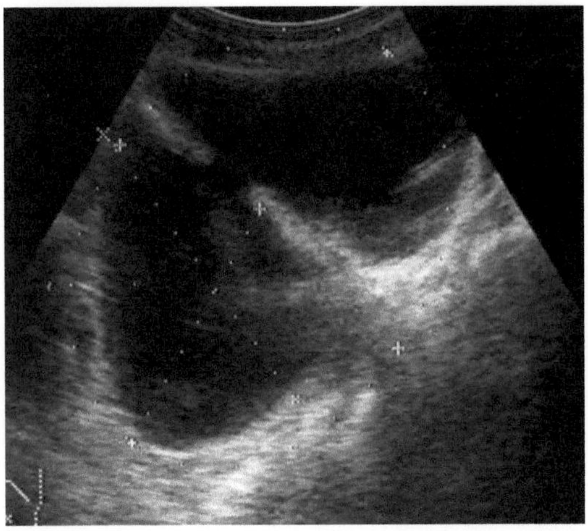

Fig. 3.3 Transabdominal ultrasonogram of the urinary bladder. A large urinary bladder diverticulum is seen (*marked with crosses*) with capacity comparable to the capacity of the urinary bladder. A short and narrow anastomosis is sharply detected which is the diverticulum neck (After Moskalyov [21])

Also the following rarer UBD complications are described: acute urine retention, acute renal failure, and urinary stasis with consequent tumoral degeneration. It is believed that the mucosa of the diverticulum is more subject to metaplasia which results from stasis of urine and a chronic infection. According to data by a number of authors, malignant tumors develop in 3–7 % of UBD [12–17].

In rare cases of UBD, *acute abdomen* symptoms and presentations similar to acute appendicitis may arise. In the literature, several cases of spontaneous diverticula rupture are described which caused development of urinary peritonitis [18, 19].

3.4 Diagnostic Imaging

The methods used for diverticula visualization and diagnosis confirmation are ultrasonography, ascending and descending cystography, computer-aided tomography, and magnetic resonance imaging [6, 20].

Urinary bladder ultrasonography is one of the leading methods of diverticula diagnostics which displays an echo-free outpouching that protrudes outside the urinary bladder outlines (Figs. 3.3, 3.4, and 3.5).

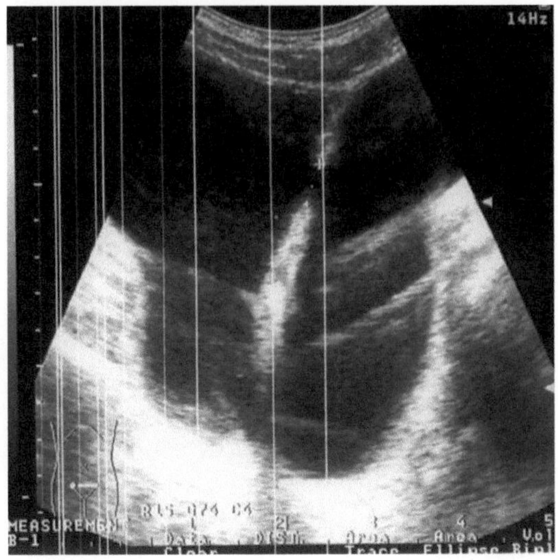

Fig. 3.4 Transabdominal ultrasonogram. The diverticulum is equal to the urinary bladder in size. Described as a two-chamber urinary bladder (After Moskalyov [21])

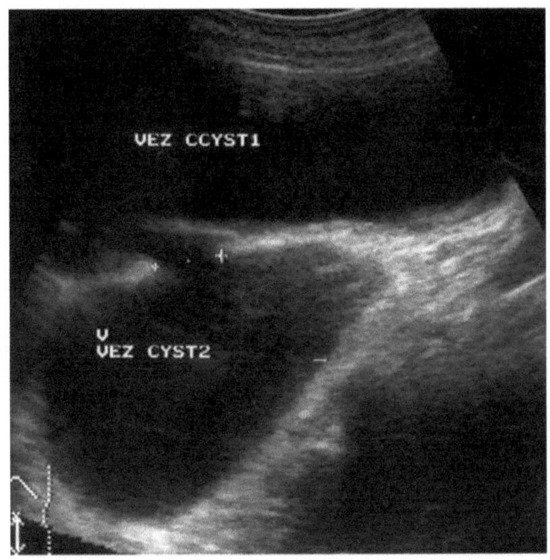

Fig. 3.5 Transabdominal ultrasonogram. Urinary bladder diverticulum is marked as VES CYST2. The diverticulum neck can be seen clearly (After Moskalyov [21])

The method allows to assess the size and localization of the diverticulum and its neck, and examination during and after urination helps to assess condition of the diverticulum wall. One of the main parameters assessed during ultrasound examination is determination of residual urine both in the diverticulum cavity and in the urinary bladder cavity. In the postsurgical period, the

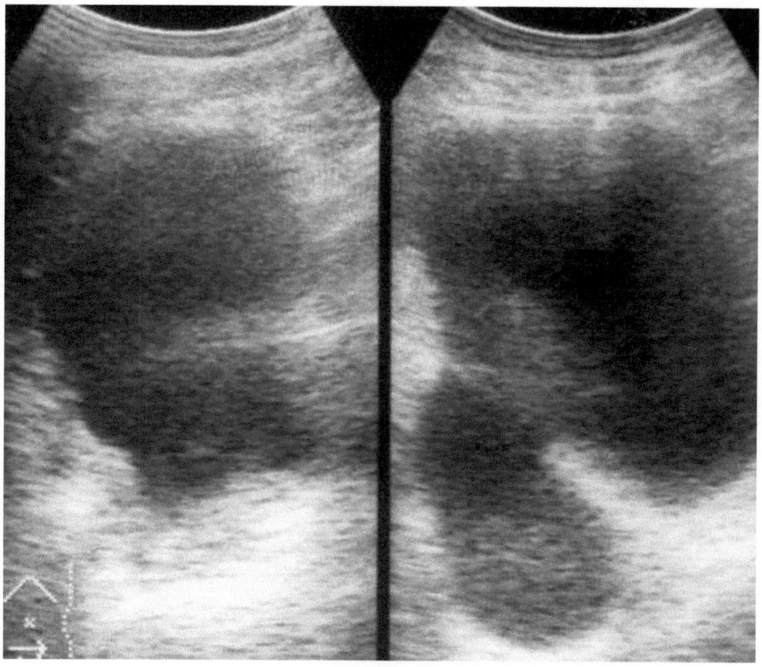

Fig. 3.6 Transabdominal ultrasonogram. Status after transurethral incision of the neck of a urinary bladder diverticulum. A diverticulum is seen which is connected with the urinary bladder by means of a wide anastomosis (After Moskalyov [21])

method is helpful for assessing effectiveness of treatment and condition of the diverticula which have undergone surgery (Fig. 3.6).

During examination it is important to reveal the diverticulum neck to differentiate it from the accumulation of liquid not related to the urinary bladder (Fig. 3.6). Ultrasonography in most cases also helps to define the cause of infravesical obstruction, such as benign hyperplasia and prostate cancer, neck sclerosis, stones in the urinary bladder, etc. Scanning with application of a transrectal probe may provide a more accurate information on diverticula in the rear and sidewalls of the urinary bladder, especially in those cases when tight filling of the bladder is impossible.

Excretory urography and cystography ensure a more vivid visualization of diverticula (Figs. 3.7 and 3.8).

In view of the fact that during direct radiography examination the diverticulum shadow may overlap the urinary bladder shadow, a multiple-view cystography or cineradiographic control is required. Retrograde and excretory cystography have almost the same information value. The latter is more preferable as it is less invasive and

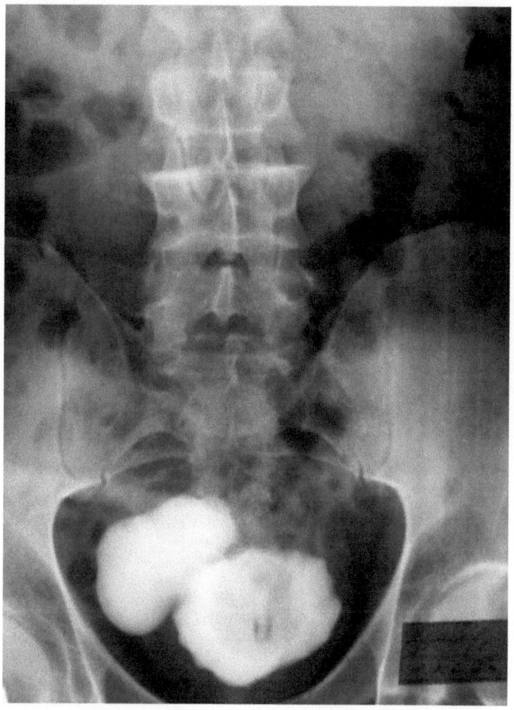

Fig. 3.7 Descending cystogram. Visible urinary bladder with a sharp irregular outline which is connected by means of a wide short neck with a urinary bladder diverticulum located in the right sidewall

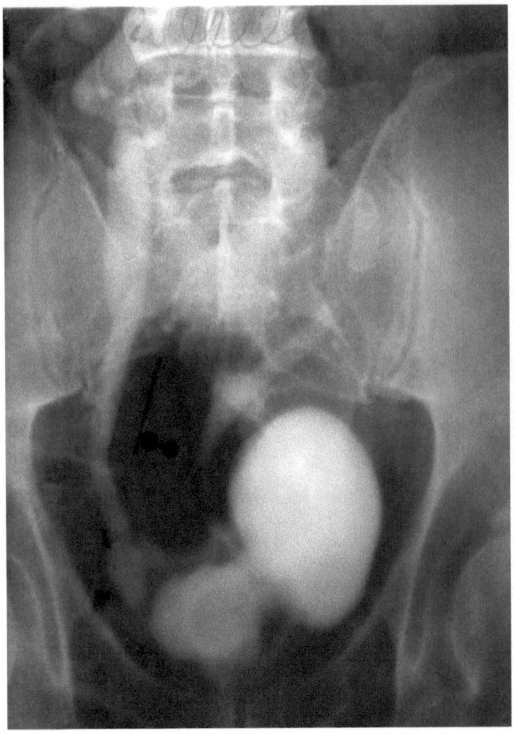

Fig. 3.8 Excretory urography with descending cystography. A big diverticulum in the left wall of the urinary bladder connected with the bladder by means of a wide neck and complicated with right-sided ureterectasia

provides a possibility to examine the condition of the upper urinary tract. In some cases, excretory urography and descending cystography are necessary in order to define the condition of the juxtavesical and intramural parts of the ureter and their relation with the diverticulum.

One of the factors which causes development of *secondary diverticula or pseudodiverticula* of the urinary bladder is a ureteral stricture which has been existing for a long time and was not treated efficiently. We observed such a case in a 49-year-old patient with a stricture in the membranous part of the urethra. The patient had suffered from that condition for more than 10 years and got repeated urethra bouginage which provided only a temporary effect (Figs. 3.9, 3.10, 3.11, 3.12, and 3.13).

Ascending cystourethrography provides more information on the condition of the bladder neck and the rear urethra which may be necessary for defining the cause of an infravesical obstruction; however, this method is rarely used nowadays due its invasive nature.

Cystography also allows to evaluate the degree of filling and voiding of the diverticulum that contributes to indirect estimation of the degree of hypotonus of the diverticulum wall.

X-ray computer-aided tomography (*CAT*) *and magnetic resonance imaging* (*MRI*) provide the most comprehensive detailing of the diverticulum, especially its neck, and display well the relation between the diverticulum and surrounding organs and tissues. These methods also ensure a better visualization of the diverticulum tumors. These methods are preferable for large diverticula in the urinary bladder when cystography is little informative due to dilution of the contrast medium and sonography—due to the reverberation effect (Figs. 3.14, 3.15, 3.16, 3.17, 3.18, 3.19, and 3.20).

Cystoscopy is one of the main methods of UBD diagnostics which should be applied in the final stage of examination as it can fill in all information gaps related to selection of a treatment method. Cystoscopy serves to assess the degree of the diverticulum neck narrowing; define the diverticulum capacity, the condition of mucosa, and connection between the diverticulum and the ureteral orifices; as well as to discover tumors and stones in the diverticulum. Before the diverticulum neck incision is performed, examination of the diverticulum cavity may be difficult in some patients due to the narrow neck. This situation hinders the introduction of an instrument into the diverticulum cavity, and in case it is possible, the instrument movement range may not be sufficient. According to a number of authors, cystoscopy is not always an accurate diagnostic method since the diverticulum orifice can be not visible due to concomitant cystitis and edema of the urinary bladder mucosa [22, 23].

Uroflowmetry does not provide information on the diverticulum presence and condition, but it is helpful in detecting the presence and degree of infravesical obstruction and evaluation of the necessary correction.

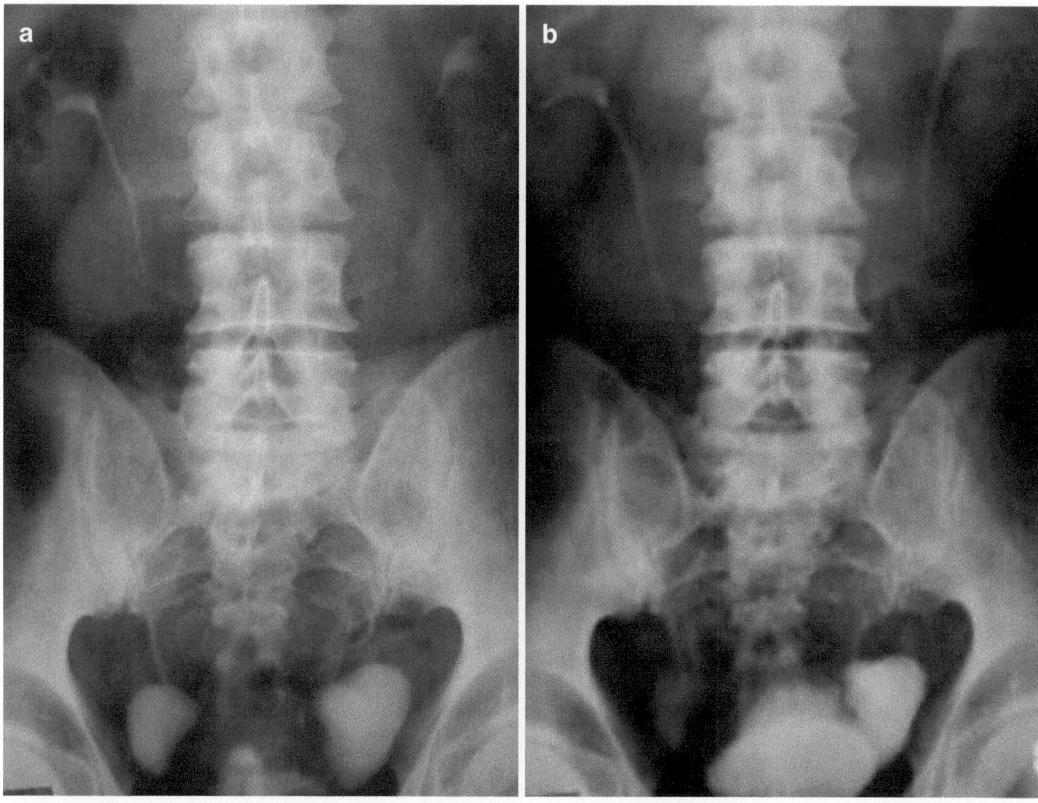

Fig. 3.9 (**a**, **b**) Excretory urograms in the 35th and 60th min (in the vertical position) in case of multiple urinary bladder diverticula

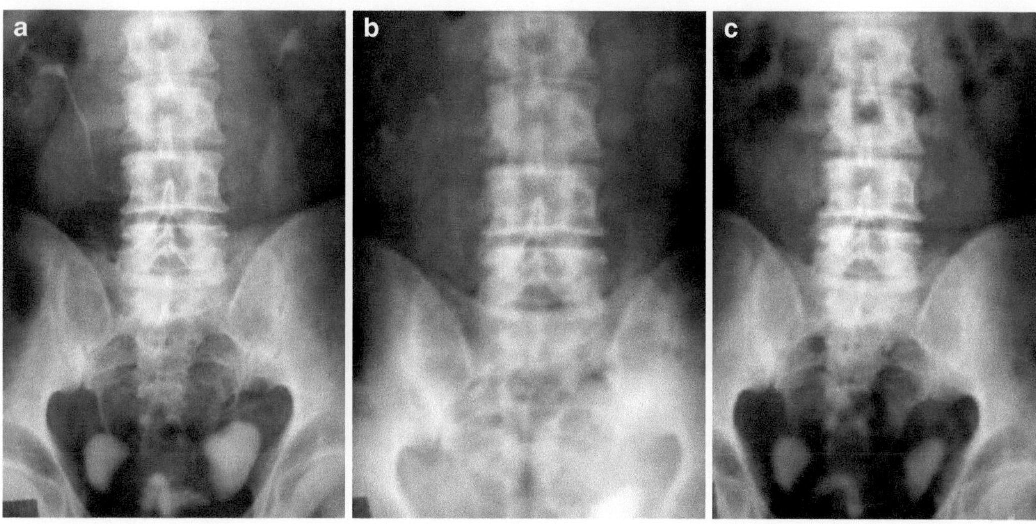

Fig. 3.10 (**a–c**) Excretory urograms in the 10th and 11th min (in the vertical position) and an overall radiogram of the same patient in 6 h

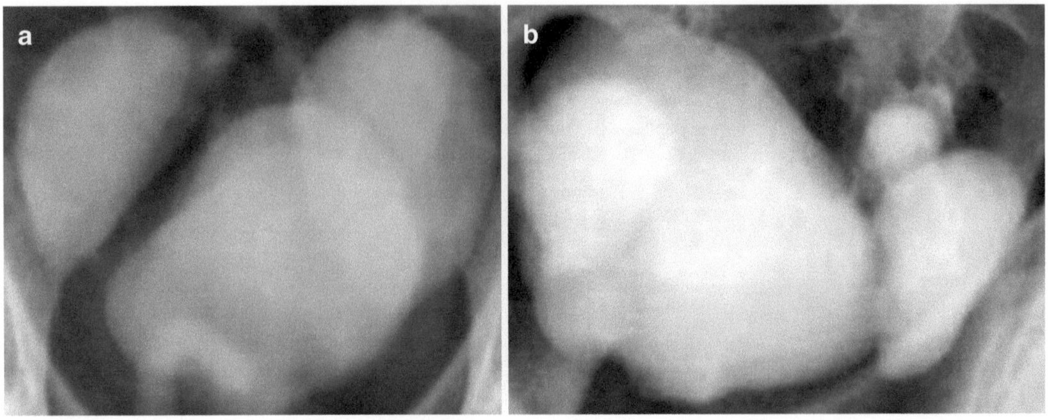

Fig. 3.11 (**a**, **b**) Three large diverticula of the urinary bladder in antegrade cystograms of the same patient which were made through a cystostomic tube

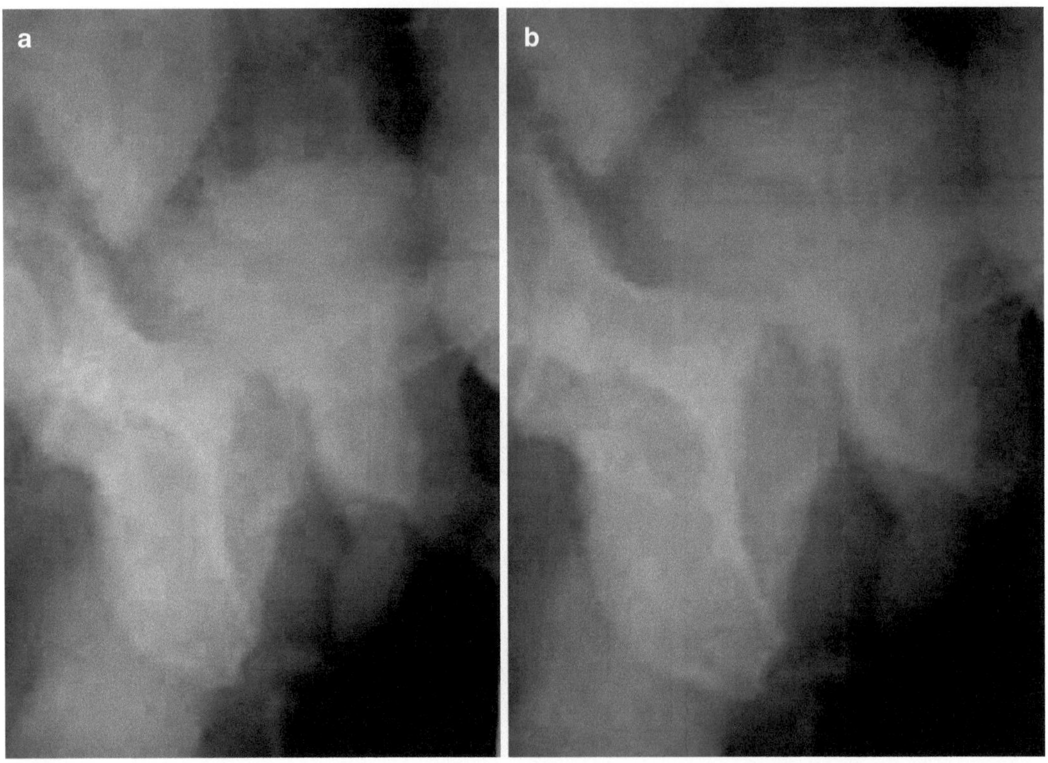

Fig. 3.12 (**a**, **b**) Voiding descending cystourethrograms of the same patient made during urination under cineradiographic monitoring—filling of large diverticula of the urinary bladder and a stricture of the urethra in the membranous part about 0.2 cm long

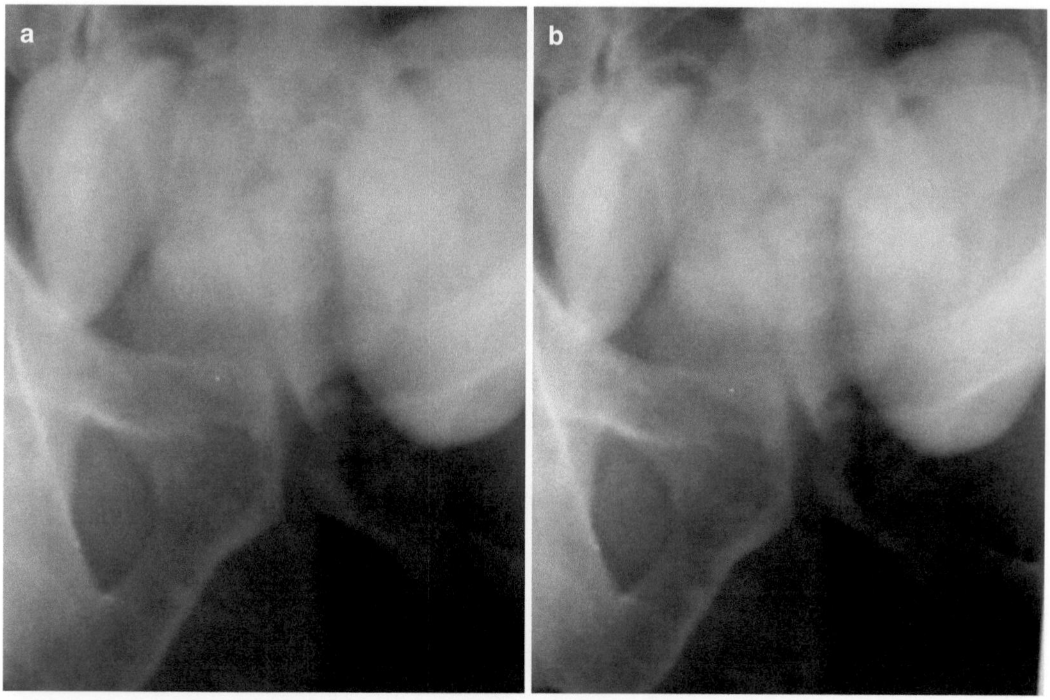

Fig. 3.13 (**a**, **b**) Voiding descending cystourethrograms of the same patient made upon completion of urination under cineradiographic monitoring—maximum filling of diverticula in the sidewalls of the urinary bladder on the left and on the right

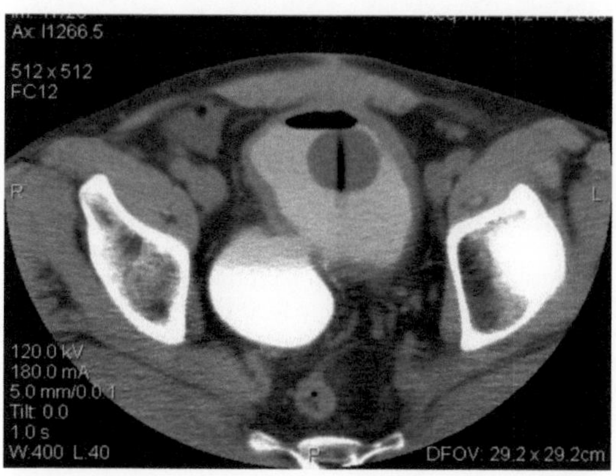

Fig. 3.14 Computer-aided tomography of the urinary bladder. Two rounded formations with sharp irregular outlines are visible, a suprapubic drainage is installed in one of them (the urinary bladder, an inflated balloon of Foley catheter is visible), and the other formation (the diverticulum) contains contrast medium. Also the narrow neck of the diverticulum and surrounding organs and tissues are well visible (After Moskalyov [21])

3.5 Treatment of the Urinary Bladder Diverticula

Usually no treatment is required in case the diverticulum is small and asymptomatic.

Conservative measures, such as lavage of the urinary bladder cavity with antiseptics and drainage of the urinary bladder, provide only a temporary relief and are justified either as preoperative preparation or as palliative treatment for patients in bad or debilitated condition that have contraindications to surgery.

There are various types and methods of surgical treatment for diverticula. Nowadays conventional open surgeries, as well as endoscopic surgeries (transurethral, laparoscopic, retroperitoneoscopic), are performed. It must be noted that the only radical method for the treatment of

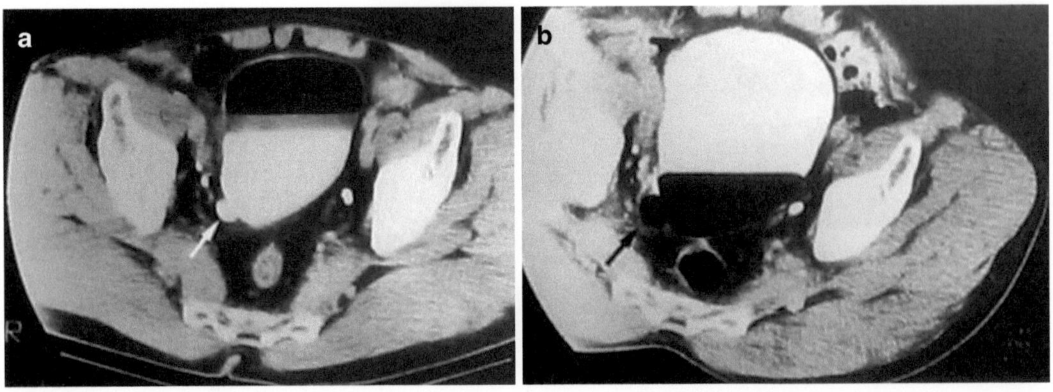

Fig. 3.15 A small urinary bladder diverticulum in a 78-year-old man: (**a**) In the CA tomogram, against double opacification of the urinary bladder, with the patient lying faceup, a small diverticulum filled with the contrast medium is visible, and the diverticulum is located on the right rear wall of the urinary bladder (*arrow*). It is specially noted that the diverticulum overlaps the ureterovesical segment. (**b**) In the left oblique view of CA tomogram, a diverticulum is visible which is filled with air (*arrow*) (After Kim et al. [20])

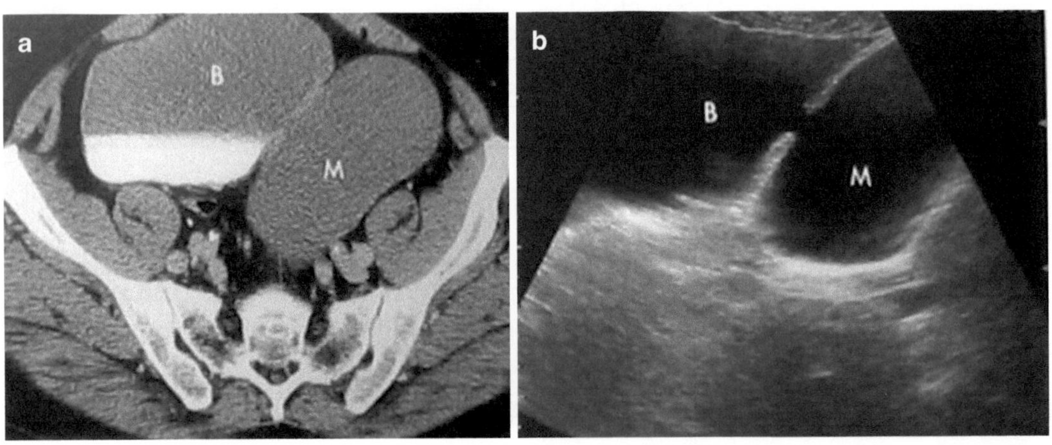

Fig. 3.16 A large urinary bladder diverticulum in a 67-year-old man: (**a**) In CA tomogram with contrast enhancement, a cystous formation (*M*) is visible in the left half of the pelvis cavity which is adjacent to the rear sidewall of the urinary bladder (*B*). A narrow channel is presumably present between the urinary bladder and the formation. (**b**) USG of the pelvic cavity reveals a duct between the urinary bladder and the formation (After Kim et al. [20])

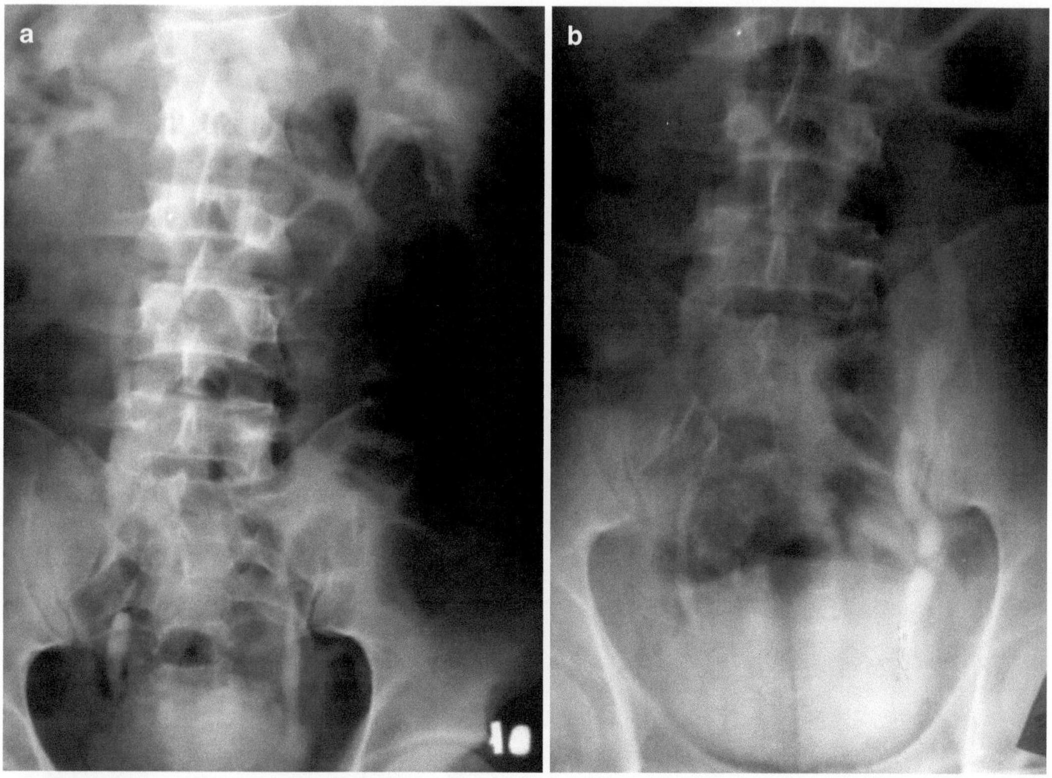

Fig. 3.17 (**a**, **b**) Excretory urograms in the 10th and 11th min with the patient standing, case of multiple congenital diverticula of the urinary bladder: (**a**) small ectasia of prevesical ureter, more on the left; (**b**) disturbed voiding with a prominent ectasia in the middle and lower third of the left ureter

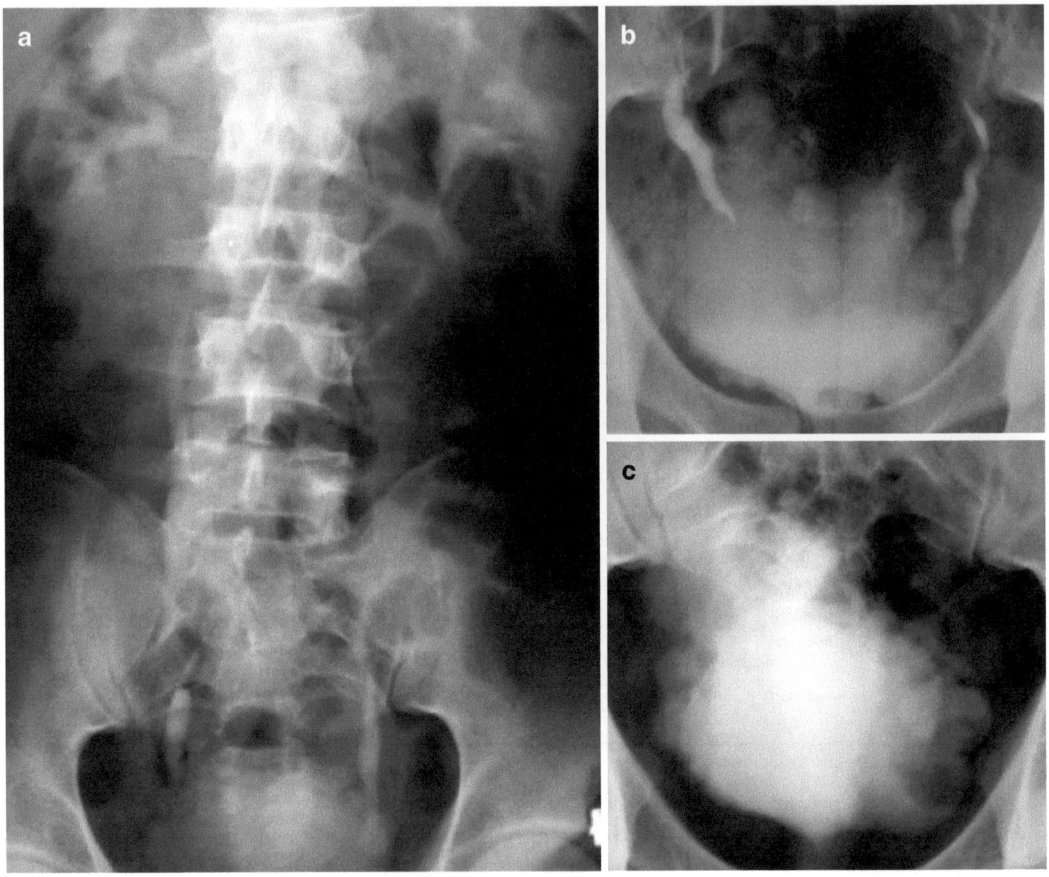

Fig. 3.18 (**a**–**c**) Excretory urogram in the 45th min and descending cystograms in the 60th and 120th min: (**a**) minor ectasia of prevesical ureters; (**b**, **c**) multiple diverticula almost along the whole perimeter of the urinary bladder

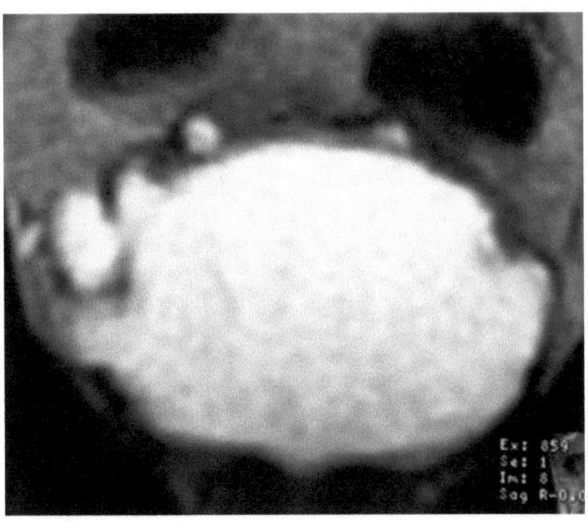

Fig. 3.19 Multiple small congenital diverticula of the urinary bladder in the coronal projection, a T2-weighted image, of the same patient

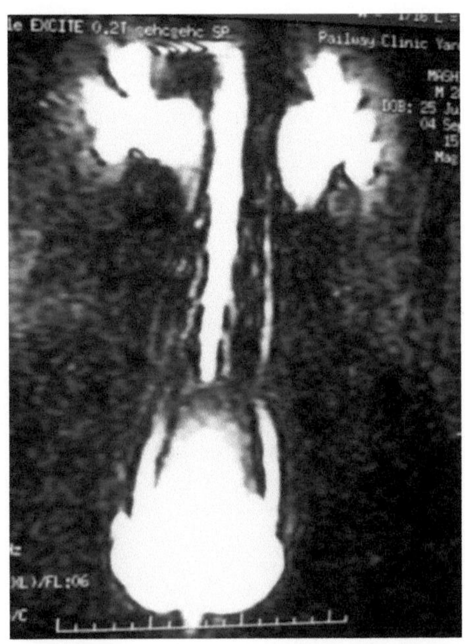

Fig. 3.20 Bilateral ureteropyelocaliectasis in the same patient in MR urograms in the coronal projection under Myelo program

the urinary bladder diverticulum is some type of diverticulectomy [24–26].

Algorithm for diagnostics of the urinary bladder diverticulum based on information value and sensitivity of various diagnostic methods (After Moskalyov [21])

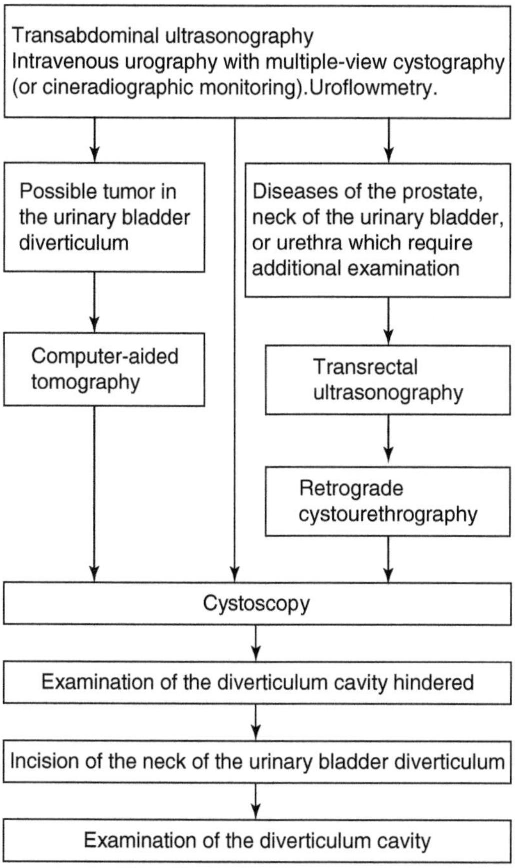

Conclusion

In summary, diagnostic imaging of the urinary bladder diverticula is relatively easy and informative both in case of USG and in case of descending cystograms, as well as when CAT and/or MRI is used. Ascending cystography in various modifications is currently used in very rare cases and is mostly of historical interest.

References

1. Abrumyants. On urinary bladder diverticula. In: 15th conference of Russian surgeons. Petrograd; 1923. p. 347–52.
2. Anchelevich VD. Pathogenesis of the urinary bladder diverticula. Urology. 1933;10(2):40–6.
3. Tyomkin IS. Urinary bladder diverticula. In: Proceedings of the 3rd All-Russia Conference of Urologists. Leningrad; 1936. p. 40–3.
4. Dunaevsky LI. Diverticula and hernias of the urinary bladder. Surgery manual in several volumes. Moscow: Meditsina; 1959. p. 329–35.
5. Clinical urology manual (under editorship of Pytel AY), vol. 2. M.: Meditsina; 1970. p. 18–21.
6. Pytel AY, Pytel YA. X-ray diagnostics in urology. M.: Meditsina; 1966. p. 347–9.
7. Ostropolskaya EA. Urinary bladder diverticula in children. Materials of reports (the First Republican Conference of Children's Surgeons of Georgia). Batumi; 1971. p. 58.
8. Blane CE, Zerin JM, Bloom DA. Bladder diverticula in children. Radiology. 1994:95;675–82.
9. Pieretti RV, Pieretti-Vanmarcke RV. Congenital bladder diverticula in children. J Pediatr Surg. 1999;34(3):468–73.
10. Lopatkin NA, Lylko AV. Abnormalities of urogenital system. Kiev: Zdorovja; 1987. p. 226–30.
11. Olsen B, Johansen TE. Urinary bladder diverticula. Tidsskr Nor Laegeforen. 1994;114:1411–3.
12. Klimenko LA. A case of undiagnosed diverticulum of the urinary bladder complicated with a stone. Some aspects of surgery of the digestive tract and retroperitoneal space. Chita: Chita State Medical Institute; 1970. p. 176–7.
13. Kim MY, Jeon YS, Suh CH, Park WH. Sarcomatoid carcinoma arising from the diverticulum of the urinary bladder dome: a difficult diagnosis with imaging. AJR Am J Roentgenol. 1999;172(5):1454–5.
14. Nuwahid F, German K, Cambell F. Carcinosarcoma in a bladder diverticulum. Urology. 1994;44:775–8.
15. Starsev VY, Karpenko AK. Results of examinations of neoplasm's arising within urinary bladder diverticulum. Eur Radiol. 2000;10(8):E25.
16. Sulaiman MN, Buchholz NP, Khan MA. Carcinoma in a bladder diverticulum: the place of diverticulectomy. Arch Ital Urol Androl. 1998;70(4):195–7.
17. Gepi Attee S, Feneley RC. Bladder diverticulectomy revisited: case report of retention of urine caused by diverticula end discussion. J Urol. 1994;152:954–5.
18. Benchekroun A, Lachkar A, Soumana A, Farih MH, Belahnech Z, Marzouk M, Faik M. Spontaneous rupture of bladder diverticulum. Apropos of a case. Ann Urol (Paris). 1998;32(6–7):367–9.
19. Iton N, Kounami T. Spontaneous rupture of a bladder diverticulum. J Urol. 1994;159:1206–13.
20. Kim SH, editor. Radiology. Illustrated uroradiology. Philadelphia: Saunders; 2003. p. 569.
21. Moskalyov AY. Transurethral endoscopic methods of treatment of the urinary bladder diverticula. Thesis for the degree of candidate of medical science, Moscow, 2003.

22. Lopatkina NA, Shevtsova IP. Urologic Surgery. Ed. Lopatkin NA, Shvetsov IP. Meditsina. Leningrad; 1986. p.210–2.
23. Netchiporenko AZ, Urbanovich VS. Transvesical excision of the urinary bladder diverticulum. Belarus Healthc. 1971;(11):73–4.
24. Adachi M, Nakada T. Transurethral treatment of bladder diverticula. Eur Urol. 1991;19:104–8.
25. Champault G, Riscalla H, Rizk N, Tchala K. Laparoscopic resection of a bladder diverticulum. Prog Urol. 1997;7:643–6.
26. Martov AG, Moskalyov AY, Guschin BL, Salyukov RV, Al-Musavi SI, Amelin AV. Endoscopic treatment of the urinary bladder diverticula. Urology. 2001;6:40–4.

4 Urethral Diverticula

Urethral diverticula (UTHD) may be found in both women and men. Their course and diagnostics depend on anatomic peculiarities of the male and female urethra (Figs. 4.1 and 4.2).

Urethra is part of the female urinary system and male urinary and genital system. The male urethra is 20 cm long and runs through both the pelvis and the penis and opens outward on its head. It has the following anatomical parts: (1) external orifice, (2) navicula, (3) penile part, (4) bulbous part, (5) membranous part, and (6) prostatic (proximal and distal parts).

The male urethra forms two curves: The first one with the curve pointing downward surrounds the pubic symphysis (*curvatura subpubica*) and the second one with the curve pointing upward is directed toward the root of the penis (*curvatura praepubica*). When seen in a urethrogram, the urethra has regular and smooth outline and has a shape of a bent strip of uneven diameter. The external sphincter of the urinary bladder divides the male urethra into two parts—the front and the rear part—each of them being divided into two parts in its turn. The front part of the urethra consists of the penile part (which runs through the penis) and bulbous part (expanded to the bulb shape), while the rear part includes the membranous part (perforating *membrana urogenitalis*) and prostatic part (surrounded by the prostate).

The female urethra is much shorter (3.0–4.0 cm) and a little wider than the male urethra, and in the urethrogram, it looks like a wide and short stripe with a regular outline. The urethra starts at the urinary bladder as an inner orifice for urine discharge, and then it runs through the urogenital diaphragm and opens as an external orifice near the pronaus in the depth of the interlabial space.

4.1 Ray Diagnostics

4.1.1 X-Ray Anatomy of the Urethra

In case of a conventional X-ray examination, images of the front and rear parts of the *male* urethra can be obtained only if two methods of introducing the contrast medium (XRCM) into the urethra lumen are combined. If the ascending or retrograde injection of XRCM is applied, the

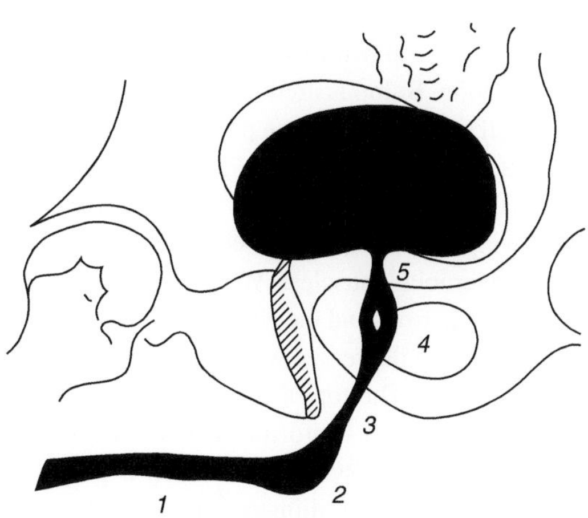

Fig. 4.1 Schematic urethrogram of a male. *1* pars pendula urethrae (cavernosa), *2* pars bulbosa, *3* pars membranacea, *4* pars prostatica (seminal hillock in the center), *5* neck of the urinary bladder (After Pytel and Pytel [1])

V.M. Builov, *Imaging of Urinary Tract Diverticula*,
DOI 10.1007/978-3-319-05383-7_4, © Springer International Publishing Switzerland 2014

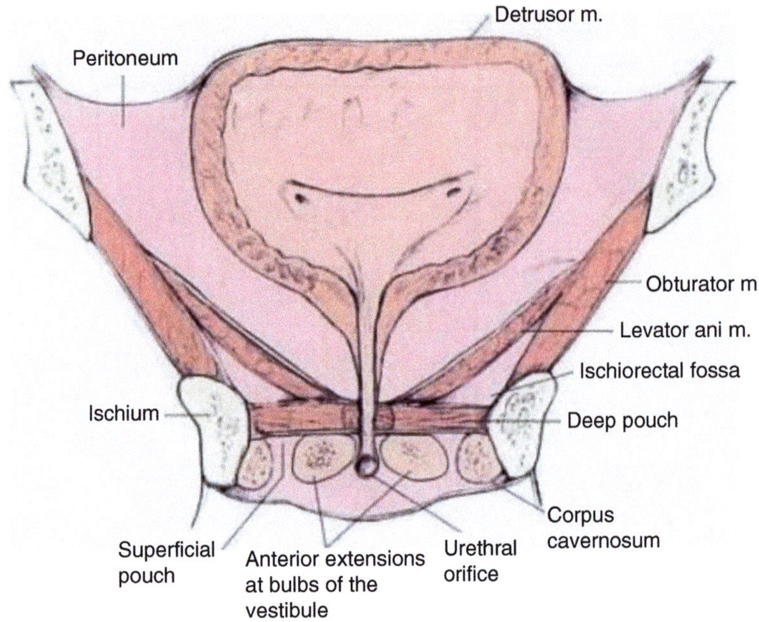

Fig. 4.2 Female urinary bladder and urethra (a schematic drawing). Front view (section). The triangle area between ureteral entrances and the inner urethral orifice is called *genitourinary region* (trigonum vesicae)

front urethra can be seen well in retrograde urethrograms. When the urinary bladder is filled with the contrast medium in the descending direction for excretory urography or when XRCM is injected in a retrograde or antegrade way into the urinary bladder, it is possible to see image of the rear urethra in the descending urethrogram during urination.

In a retrograde urethrogram, a normal front urethra of an adult male starting from the navicula and along the whole cavernous part can be traced as a strip with even parallel edges 1.0–1.5 cm wide. Bulbous urethra expands at the bottom wall and forms a curve pointing downward.

The rear urethra length is 3–4 cm. Its lumen above the external sphincter is tapered. Moderate narrowing around the cone edges is created by bulbocavernous muscles. When these muscles contract, the front and the sidewalls of this part of the urethra are depressed which may be mistaken for a stricture. The top of the tapered end of the front urethra passes into the rear urethra which upon retrograde XRCM introduction expands to a width of several millimeters and has a slight bent with incurvity in the front. The rear urethra forms a right or a little greater angle with the front urethra and extends as far as the bladder bottom.

The seminal hillock at the back wall of the prostatic urethra forms a spindle-shaped bulging. Location of the seminal hillock varies from the middle to the most distal part of the rear urethra. The upper and the lower poles of the seminal hillock pass into the urethral crest which is several millimeters wide and gradually flattens in the distal and proximal directions. The sides of the crest are supracollicularly formed by two shallow grooves which reach the neck of the bladder. Normally there is another shallow groove in the front wall of the urethra which extends from the urinary bladder to the level of the seminal hillock. All these grooves become invisible upon a significant expansion of the urethra lumen which takes place during urination.

If the urethra is unchanged, the prostatic and other paraurethral passages can be seen in retrograde urethrograms only under excessively strong pressure during XRCM introduction or through artificial blockade of the urinary bladder neck.

In case of voiding urethrography, the neck of the urinary bladder expands during urination and takes the form of a funnel. Rugae in the supracollicular part of the rear urethra disappear and its lumen becomes much larger (in an average up to 0.5 cm or more in the lateral projection on the level of the seminal hillock). Further, to the distal side from the external sphincter, the urethral lumen narrows.

During urination the rear urethra lowers due to lowering of the pelvic floor. This lowering is more prominent in the upper and rear parts of the pelvic floor which causes a displacement of the urinary bladder neck and of the upper part of the prostatic urethra downward and backward, and the rear urethra takes a more horizontal position. It must be kept in mind that the degree of the rear urethra repositioning depends also on the degree of the abdominal pressure increase during urination.

The female urethra is 3.0–4.0 cm long; the sphincter part takes two thirds of its length while one third is the intercavernous part. The sphincter part corresponds to the rear male urethra. In place of the male prostate, the female system contains a great number of paraurethral glands which are located mostly in the middle third of the urethra. Similar to the prostate glands, the female paraurethral glands are partly surrounded by nonstriated muscles. The external sphincter surrounds the urethra on the rear side in a horseshoe shape, merges with the retrourethral tissue (median lobe) and partly surrounds the vagina. The mucosa of both female and male urethras has longitudinal rugae which are well seen after moderate feeling of the urethra with a liquid XRCM.

UTHD, as all other diverticula, are divided into *congenital and acquired ones.*

Congenital UTHD are rare and have the form of saccular outpouchings of the rear wall connected by a narrow duct with the urethra, and like all other true diverticula, they comprise the same layers as the urethra.

Most often UTHD are localized in the front part of the urethra. The congenital UTHD diameter may be from 1 to 5–6 cm. These must be differentiated from *the acquired UTHD* which often appear after a trauma, including traumas of iatrogenic etiology, due to the development of the urethra stricture and presence of stones and foreign objects in it. In addition to that, the development of an acquired UTHD is related with paraurethral abscesses and festering cysts.

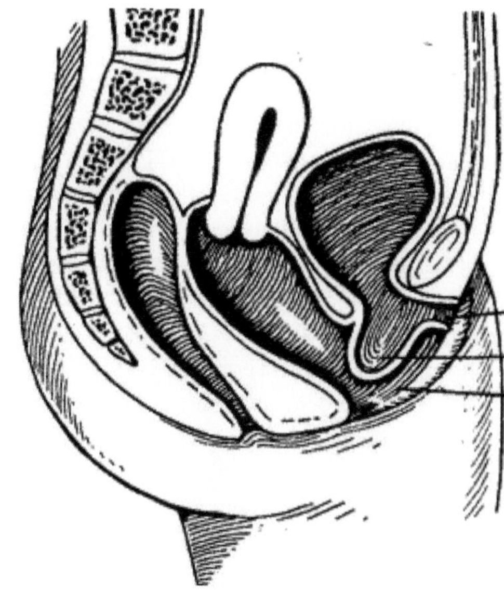

Fig. 4.3 Schematic drawing of the urethral diverticulum: *1* diverticulum, *2* external urethral orifice, *3* vaginal orifice (After Mazhbits [2]

4.2 Female Urethra Diverticula

The urethral diverticulum is an outpouching of the rear wall which is connected with the urethral duct by means of a fistulous tract. This opening may vary in size and location; it may be located in any area between the external and internal urethral orifices; however, its most common location is the front part of the urethral duct (Figs. 4.1 and 4.3).

4.2.1 Etiology, Localization, Pathogenesis, and Pathophysiology of UTHD

Based on literature evidence, paraurethral cysts and/or UTHD are found up to 1–6 % [2–6] more often in women at the age of 20 to 60 years. As noted by [7–14], although, based on the literature, UTHD frequency rate is 1–6 %, these data may be significantly lowered. According to Mazhbits [2], lately an increase of number of female patients with this disease is reported which may be related both with a greater number of patients who got inadequate treatment of sexually transmitted infections and with the widespread occurrence of various hygiene preparations based on soap. This causes obstruction of excretory ducts of paraurethral glands, development of inflammation, and, a as a result, development of a paraurethral cyst and/or UTHD.

As noted by [16–18], some authors consider UTHD a rare disease in female patients and classify it as anecdotal evidence. Other authors on the contrary report spreading of this disease and find it in 2–3 % women [19].

In the opinion of Pereverzev [18], UTHD is rarely found in women, and according to some authors, its frequency is 0.6–6 % among adults [1, 2]. Approximately the same statistics has been reported during the recent years, 1–5 % [3]. In accordance with this study which was carried out for 18 years and included investigation of the causes of recurrent infection in 863 women, true diverticula of the female urethra were found in 16 patients (2 %), ureterocele in 27 patients (3 %), and paraurethral cysts in 24 patients (3 %).

Existence of the female urethra diverticulum was described for the first time by W. Hey in 1805 [4]; however that nosologic unit was rarely defined until 1930 year, when occasional reports of this pathology started to appear. The general understanding and diagnostics of the disease have been improving since 1950 when urethrography with positive pressure was suggested. Thus H.J. Davis and K.W. Telinde published data on 121 female patient with UTHD which exceeded the number of such patients discovered for the preceding 60 years [22].

In 1970 an analysis of results of diagnostics and treatment of 120 UTHD in women was published which was carried out already in one clinic [23]. UTHD are found in women mostly at the age of 20–60 years (on average in 40-year-old patients), although it must be noted that they occur more often than they are diagnosed. If a histologic examination reveals unstriated muscles, it means that the UTHD has the congenital nature. However the majority of UTHD are acquired.

Numerous clinical observations confirm that UTHD are found at locations of paraurethral glands; however theories of UTHD pathogenesis have been actively debated for more than a century. Theories of UTHD formation are mostly focused on the following aspect: whether they are acquired or congenital. If UTHD are congenital, can they result from infections, childbearing, or even from iatrogeny? Proofs for the congenital nature of the disease lose their ground in view of the fact that UTHD are rarely found in girls. Thus during examination of 121 female patient which was carried out by the abovementioned authors [17], not a single case of the disease was diagnosed in patients under 20 years. Only 6.5 % of those patients developed symptoms before they reached the age of 20. Observations under analysis [17] confirm that the disease is congenital. The evidence is based on observations which revealed the location of diverticula in the area where atropic ureter is joining the urethra. Diverticula are located in the areas containing residual Gartner's ducts, and some female patients were treated for UTHD containing cloacogenic rudiments.

At the same time there are judgments supporting the acquired UTHD genesis. At the beginning of the previous century, a birth trauma was considered to be the cause of their formation. From the pathogenetic point of view, it was explained as follows: The layer of the inner urethral muscles was ruptured under the pressure created by the fetus head or obstetric forceps which resulted in the formation of a hernia or a diverticulum. However further studies provided a reliable evidence that UTHD may occur in nonporous patients as well; thus based only on that fact, the hypothesis of the disease of acquired nature was rejected.

More acceptable are explanations stating that recurrent infections and obstruction of paraurethral glands cause development of suburethral cysts. These cysts may rupture spontaneously and break into the urethra lumen. Continuous irritation with urine which is retained in the cavity of this formation during each urination may finally result in epithelization and formation of a permanent diverticulum. Nowadays this explanation is accepted by majority of researchers who regard UTHD as an acquired disease of infectious etiology. There are reasons to believe that paraurethral glands get infected by the normal vaginal flora. The most often grown cultures are *Escherichia coli* and other gram-negative bacteria such as *Staphylococcus aureus* and

Streptococcus faecalis. Nowadays it is believed that a urethral infection affecting paraurethral glands may cause formation of diverticula; however more often the leading role in the disease etiology is attributed to gonorrhea [18–21].

Many other possible UTHD causes were suggested: a birth trauma; high intravesical pressure during urination caused by closure and spasm of the external sphincter in neurologic patients, instrumental injuries, stones in a ureter, and also urethral strictures; and performance of urethral and vaginal surgeries which may be complicated with incomplete regeneration or a secondary infection. There are indications of a possible etiologic role of endometriosis, although among 46 observations of diverticula in the female urethra, only one case of endometriosis was reported [25]. Congenital factors may be present, including defects of Gartner's ducts, a faulty union of primordial folds, the presence of cell rests, as well as wolffian ducts or vaginal cysts opening into the urethra. Experiments made by Hoffman [24] who got wax patterns of inflamed urethra revealed orifices of paraurethral glands in its lumen. These experiments confirm the concept of transformation of a suburethral infectious inflammation into abscess which is later covered with epithelium. Paraurethral glands get inflamed and block and later they break into the urethra creating linking channels between the diverticulum and the urethral lumen. According to microscopic studies, paraurethral glands can be found along the greatest part of the urethra (the rear and lateral location mostly), and most of them open in the distal part of the urethra. They represent a complicated system of tubuloalveolar structures and their number may be more than 30. Skene glands which are the largest of the paraurethral glands are emptied into the external orifice of the urethra and are often considered separately.

Paraurethral glands are tubuloalveolar structures which are mostly found in the distal two thirds of the urethra and open in the same area. In the macroscopic scale, paraurethral glands vary from simple saccular structures to complicated brachiferous structures. Their inflammation and disturbance of drainage into the urethra may also promote formation of diverticula in the distal part of the urethra. Sometimes the diverticula may have an extremely proximal location; in very rare cases they spread under the neck of the urinary bladder and the area of the vesical triangle [26].

Acquired UTHD develop from inflamed and blocked paraurethral glands which are usually found in the submucosal layer of the spongy tissue of the distal two thirds of the urethra. Cysts and abscesses gradually grow in size due to recurrent inflammations and obstructed ducts of paraurethral glands. Initially the growth results from displacement of the spongy vascular tissue and muscles of the urethra. The further growth weakens the urethra lining which leads to formation of a hernial bulging and detachment of two fascial layers of the urethropelvic ligament. In most cases, the diverticular sac expands to the back of the urethra which results in the development of a typical soft cystous formation on the front wall of the vagina. Not uncommon is the diverticulum expansion to the side which may be accompanied by a less prominent increase in volume and a greater detachment and separation of the vaginal and abdominal layers of urethropelvic ligaments. Less frequent is the diverticulum expansion to the front of the urethra, and still less frequent, it surrounds the urethra in the shape of a horseshoe. UTHD can be small and large, solitary and multiple, or multilocular. Finally the diverticulum contents break into the urethra lumen and a connection between the urethra and diverticulum appears. In some cases it breaks into the vagina causing formation of a urethrovaginal fistula. This concept is especially important for understanding surgical methods used for resection of the urethral diverticulum.

As noted by Pushkar and Anisimov [3], the term *paraurethral cyst* is not used in the overseas literature, and those conditions which are referred to and regarded as the paraurethral cyst in Russia are treated there only as a stage of UTHD pathogenesis.

4.2.2 Clinical Picture

About 20 % of UTHD are asymptomatic. In case clinical presentations are observed, the most typical complaint is urine dribbling after urination. There is a pictorial description which should be kept in mind during urethral diverticulum diagnostics, namely, *three Ds*: dysuria (disturbed urination), dribbling (intermittent flow of urine or dripping), and dyspareunia (sexual disorders) [3, 11–15]. This classical trilogy is typical for the urethral diverticulum. Sometimes urine has a putrefactive odor. Infection of UTHD causes painful urination (dysuria) and pains in the perineum and increase of the residual urine volume. Clinical symptoms in case of UTHD may vary from weak and occasional discomfort to strong pain and pronounced retention of urine in case of an acute infection. However in majority of patients, nonspecific irritative symptoms develop which are typical for the lower urinary tract in case of cystitis. Apart from the classical trilogy which is characteristic of UTHD, they may include the following symptoms: uroclepsia, hematuria, recurrent infections of the urinary tract, and urine retention. UTHD complications include stasis of urine and development of an infection in UTHD that creates ideal conditions for lithogenesis in some patients.

Mazhbits [2] suggested the following stages of UTHD course which lead to lithogenesis: (1) First is catarrhal diverticulitis which often proceeds without any clinical presentations. In such cases the cloudy urine which comes out of the diverticulum contains a small amount of epithelial cell and leucocytes. (2) Second is acute purulent diverticulitis with frank clinical presentations which is often complicated with inflammation of the rear urethra and the vesical triangle. Such a diverticulum has a swollen mucosa with a pronounced injection of blood vessels in some areas. The purulent contents consist of leucocytes, epithelial cells, erythrocytes, and a large number of bacteria. (3) Third is ulcerated diverticulitis, which often results in perforation due to destruction and thinning if the urethral wall tissue (G. Z. Gorovits). (4) Fourth is urethral diverticulum containing a single or multiple stones. This kind of diverticulitis could be described as calculous. The author described resection of the UTHD from which a stone was removed, 2×3 cm, with rough surface and hard texture, which caused insupportable pain during and after urination. He also provided observations by Mazhbits [2], who had described an extremely rare observation of the urethral diverticulum that contained 24 small faceted stones of various sizes in its cavity. Analysis revealed that they consisted of a mixture of phosphates, triple phosphates, and magnesium with a small amount of urates and carbonates. Organic matrix consists of protein. D. N. Atabekov diagnosed stones in diverticula in 2 of 13 patients. Stones were discovered in 7 out of 17 patients with diverticula operated by A. M. Mazhbits. A key sign of UTHD can be the presence of recurrent urinary tract infections in the anamnesis which were resistant to antibacterial therapy. A number of other symptoms (namely, presence of a tumorlike formation in the vagina, discharge from the urethra, painful ambulation) depend on localization of the diverticulum orifice. Urine retention, which occurs rarely, usually results from the presence of large proximal diverticula that obstruct and block the urinary bladder neck. These diverticula develop due to narrowing after recurrent infections. There are rare reports of formation of stones in diverticular cavity, including giant stones [12, 34]. Usually none of the symptoms described is proportionate to the diverticulum size. Thus large diverticula are often not sensed by patients, while small UTHD in case of an active infection may have very strong symptoms. Chronical complaints do not bear a uniform character; long periods of spontaneous remission are not uncommon. In addition to that, a carcinoma of the urethra may be defined in the diverticulum [6–10].

Signs of UTHD During Physical Examination: The typical sign discovered during physical examination is a palpable mass lesion which is found under the urethra by vaginal touch. Pressure on UTHD causes an acute pain during urination. If the diverticulum is located in the rear urethra, the latter can be palpated through the straight intestine or by vaginal touch in women [2]. In some cases it is identified by purulent discharge from the urethra upon compression. However often no signs are discovered and UTHD is not diagnosed during physical examination.

4.2.3 Diagnostics

UTHD diagnostics comprises conventional examination methods: anamnesis taking, objective examination, cystourethroscopy, urethrography, and, during the recent years, SCT urethrography, as well as MRI and MR urethrography.

Many authors emphasize that in UTHD diagnostics feature a high degree of suspicion since UTHD are not uncommon in women.

Visualization and palpation of the front wall of the vagina reveal a soft tissue formation 2–3 cm in size, sometimes up to 6 cm. A giant UTHD which comes from the distal urethra may prolapse from the distal urethra simulating uterine prolapse.

Upon light compression of that formation with fingers, urine or purulent substance comes out from the external orifice of the urethra. While examining the urethra, it is very important to define the position of the proximal urethra and the urinary bladder neck.

In case a diverticulum is suspected in a female urethra based on anamnesis and the objective examination, an additional examination must be performed in order to detect the size and localization of the diverticulum [2, 17, 26, 27, 29, 40]. According to [15, 16], in most cases a correct diagnosis for paraurethral cysts can be made by means of visual examination and palpation. At the same time one should keep in mind the necessity of differential diagnostics with tumors of the front wall of the vagina, urethrocystocele, paravesical (Gartner's) cysts, as well as UTHD. The concept which exists in a number of domestic publications differentiates the paraurethral cyst from the UTHD, unlike the concept which is more popular in the overseas literature according to which the paraurethral cyst is only a stage of the UTHD development.

In order to diagnose a paraurethral cyst and/or urethral diverticulum, Pushkar and Anisimov [3] suggest the following plan for examination of female patients: (1) examination of patients on the gynecological chair, (2) USG including transvaginal ultrasonography, (3) urethral profilometry, (4) urethrocystoscopy, (5) X-ray methods of examination, and (6) magnetic resonance imaging (MRI) with an endorectal coil. *Gynecological examination* is the primary method of examining female patients with paraurethral formations. It helps to determine shape, consistency, displaceability, painfulness of the paraurethral formation, and its connection with the urethra. Often by applying pressure to the formation, it is possible to discover discharge of a turbid secretion from the urethra which may indicate a connection of the latter with the urethra. Based on examination results, it is possible to make a diagnosis in case of typical presentations of a paraurethral cyst (Figs. 4.4 and 4.5).

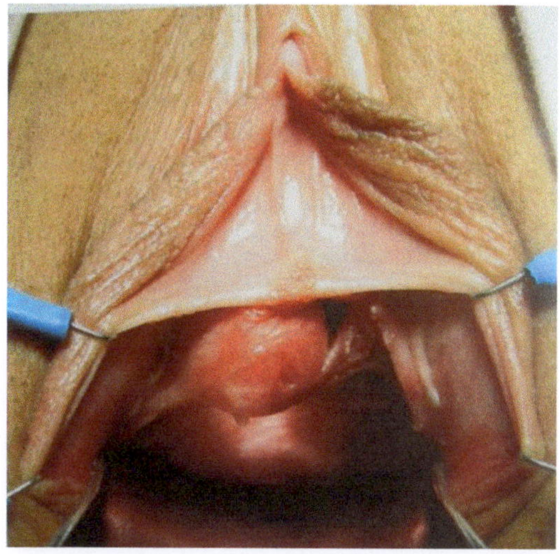

Fig. 4.4 A photo of a paraurethral cyst (After Pushkar and Anisimov [3])

USG, preferably with a transvaginal probe, at the frequency of 6.5 MHz, allows to define the relation between the paraurethral cyst and the urethra. Changing the position of the scan plane in relation to the urethra sometimes helps to reveal communication of the cyst cavity with the urethral lumen in the form of a narrow non-echogenic fistulous tract; however it is by far not always possible due to infiltrative and fibrous changes around the urethra (Figs. 4.4 and 4.6).

Urethral profilometry is used to define the location of the UTHD orifice and differential diagnostics of paraurethral cysts and UTHD. In many cases during profilometry, an increase of the maximum intraurethral pressure at the level of the formation is detected.

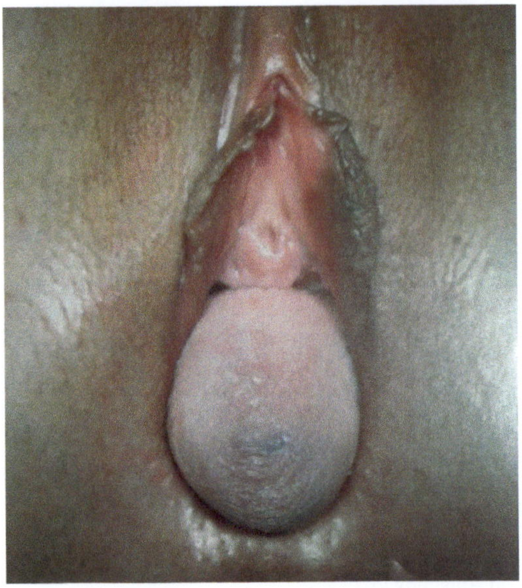

Fig. 4.5 A photo of a paraurethral cyst (After Pushkar and Anisimov [3])

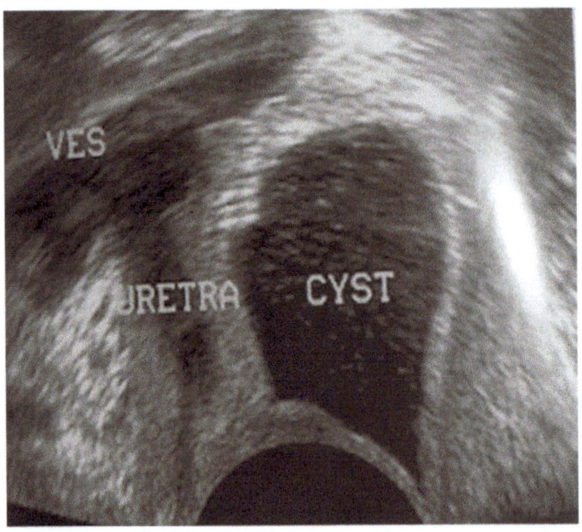

Fig. 4.6 Ultrasound image of a paraurethral cyst (After Pushkar and Anisimov [3])

During urethrocystoscopy for a better urethra visualization, it is recommended to carry out the examination against a continuous injection of a sterile liquid into the urethra via a cystoscope; this provides straightening of urethral rugae and aids visualization of a possible UTHD orifice. In addition to that, the inner urethra orifice is pressed with a finger in order to stretch the diverticulum to facilitate its visualization. Massage of the urethra during examination may provide a discharge of a turbid contents form the diverticulum orifice; however the UTHD orifice cannot always be observed directly. With a wide UTHD orifice, it is sometimes possible to examine the diverticulum cavity, where in 5 % of cases lithogenesis is observed [6]. Also there are described cases of malignant changes of the mucosa which lines the diverticulum cavity and development of a tumor in the diverticulum [8–10].

Such method of X-ray examination as voiding cystourethrography enables differential diagnostics between UTHD and paraurethral cyst. Prior to voiding cystography, the preliminary plan radiography of the pelvis must not be omitted as it can reveal stones in the UTHD cavity. Voiding cystourethrography is performed on a standing patient under cineradiographic monitoring after introduction of 250.0–300.0 ml of the contrast medium into the urinary bladder through a urethral catheter. This method may help to determine location of the UTHD and its orifice; however it is successful only in case of a relatively large diverticulum orifice.

Apart from this method, *retrograde urethrography with positive pressure in the urethra* is used for ray diagnostics of UTHD in women. This method implies filling of the urethra with one balloon blocking the external urethral orifice and the other balloon blocking the neck of the urinary bladder (Fig. 4.4). It is evident that a special catheter is required for this examination. This is the most accurate method to make a diagnosis. Methylene blue or indigo carmine can be added to the contrast medium to provide blue coloring during the subsequent urethroscopy in the UTHD cavity (Fig. 4.7).

For this examination, a special two-balloon catheter is used which is installed into the urethra so that the distal balloon is located near the neck of the urinary bladder. The distal and then the proximal balloons are inflated by injecting 30.0 ml of liquid into them. When the inflated balloons block both ends of the urethra, 5–7 ml of the contrast medium is injected via the duct which opens between the balloons; this contrast medium flows around the catheter and fills the UTHD cavity. This method of examination is

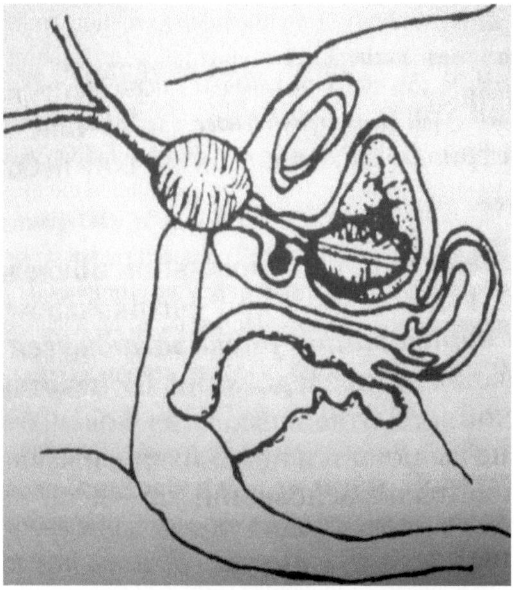

Fig. 4.7 Retrograde urethrography with positive pressure provides filling of the diverticulum (After Appell [12])

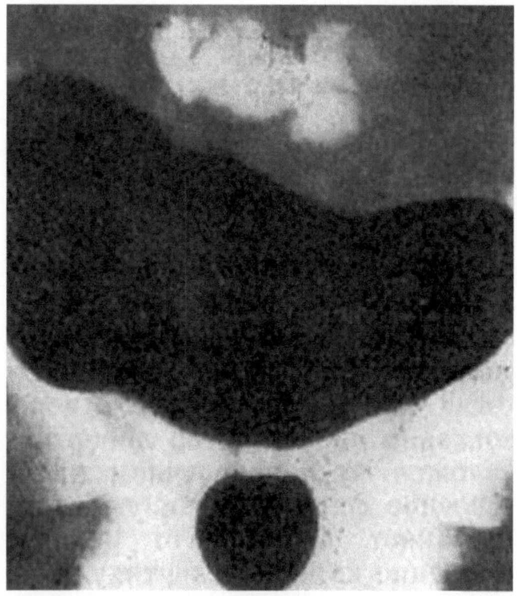

Fig. 4.8 X-ray image of a urethral diverticulum (Observation by Mazhbits [2])—simultaneous cystography and diverticulography. The urinary bladder and the diverticulum are opacified; the urinary bladder has the shape of a horseshoe, and the urethral diverticulum has a nearly round shape

much more accurate for UTHD diagnostics compared to voiding cystourethrography (Fig. 4.5). As emphasized by [17], a tight UTHD filling with contrast medium reveals the size and outline of the diverticular cavity. Nowadays that is the optimum way for diagnostics of urethral diverticula in women. During some examinations, if the diverticulum neck has a large orifice, a metal catheter can be introduced into its cavity followed by filling with a contrast medium (retrograde diverticulography). A diverticulogram provides a clear picture of the diverticulum anatomy as well as its location, shape, and size (Figs. 4.8, 4.9, and 4.10).

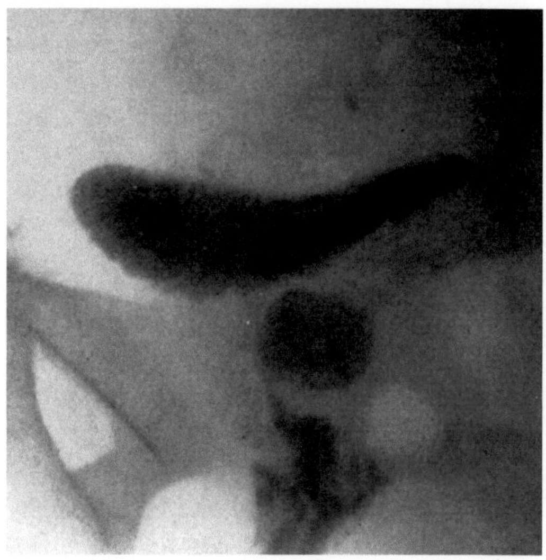

Fig. 4.9 Retrograde urethrocystogram. A cyst of a globular shape (diverticulum) which is communicating with the urethra and adjacent to its medium third and can be formally classified as an acquired urethral diverticulum (After Stepanov and Goldin [27])

4.2.3.1 Puncture Radiography of a Cyst

This method of paraurethral cyst diagnostics used to be popular before USG and MRI introduction as an X-ray method to confirm diagnosis, define the size of the cystous cavity, and clarify its location relative to the urethra and neck of the urinary bladder. Below we describe our observation as an example [28]. A 47-year-old female patient was admitted to the urological clinic with complaints of painful polyuria and repeating uroclepsia. The woman had been ill for 8 months since she developed dysuria and hematuria after an excessive exposure to cold. The patient got ambulatory treatment for acute cystitis with a

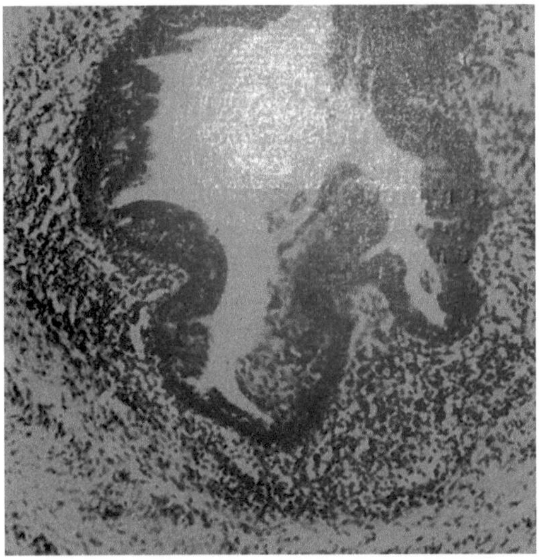

Fig. 4.10 Microphoto (the same female patient) of a wall of paraurethral cysts, coloring with hematoxylin and eosine, 80× (After Stepanov and Goldin [27])

minor effect. She was consulted by gynecologist and urologist who diagnosed her with a paraurethral cyst and recommended surgery. The patient specified the following previous diseases: influenza, angor, and trichomoniasis; she had also been under the supervision of a gynecologist for the preceding 7 years for metrofibroma and chronic adnexitis. Vulva is developed normally. During vaginal touch, a formation could be palpated in the front wall of the vagina, which was 8.0×8.0 cm in size, moderately painful, and fluctuating; when pressed, about 80.0 ml of thick greenish fetid purulence was discharged from the urethra. The formation periodically emptied and then enlarged again which was accompanied by hematuria, increase of body temperature up to 38° centigrade, and aggravation of dysuria up to acute urine retention which required urine drainage with a rubber catheter. Excretory urograms revealed no anatomic or functional changes in the kidneys and the upper urinary tract. The urinary bladder in the descending cystogram was enlarged and lifted over the pubic articulation. In the ascending cystogram, shifting of the urinary bladder upward and to the right was observed. In the puncture cystogram done under cineradiographic monitoring (the contrast media was introduced into the cyst transvaginally after its partial voiding), a multilocular formation could be seen at the level of the pubic articulation (Fig. 4.12). When the rubber catheter was introduced into the urinary bladder, a central position of the urethra relative to the formation was detected, while the formation surrounded the urethra in the shape of a horseshoe. It was recommended to remove the paraurethral cyst by surgery in 1.5–2.0 months after the elimination of inflammation. Three months later, an elective surgery was performed under general anesthesia. During a follow-up examination in 2.5 months after the surgery, the patient had no complaints and the paraurethral cyst was not found. The peculiarity of this observation was empyema of the paraurethral cyst with its recurrent expansion that caused an acute urine retention which is rarely observed in women (Fig. 4.11).

4.2.3.2 Magnetic Resonance Imaging

Nowadays the most up-to-date and efficient method of ray diagnostics in urology, including UTHD diagnostics, is magnetic resonance imaging (MRI), the only disadvantage of this method being its rather high cost.

Transurethral and transvaginal sonography may be used to characterize UTHD; however these methods have a limited visual field, unlike MRI which provides perfect contrasting of tissues and a possibility of multiplane reconstruction. This enables a detailed examination of the female urethra anatomy and clarification of the lesion degree, which is very beneficial for surgery planning. Discharge from the urethra in case of UTHD is displayed like a vivid hyperintensive signal in the T2-weighted image near or around the urethra. Upon introduction of magnetic resonance contrast media which contain gadolinium, no accumulation of gadolinium in UTHD is observed.

During recent years, MRI usage for UTHD diagnostics is increasing due to its noninvasiveness, absence of exposure of patients to radiation, and high sensitivity. MRI technology with endorectal coil is preferable. Examination is made with the urinary bladder full. The rectal coil is inserted into the straight intestine and fixed there by means of a balloon inflated with air. MRI with an endorectal coil enables a detailed study

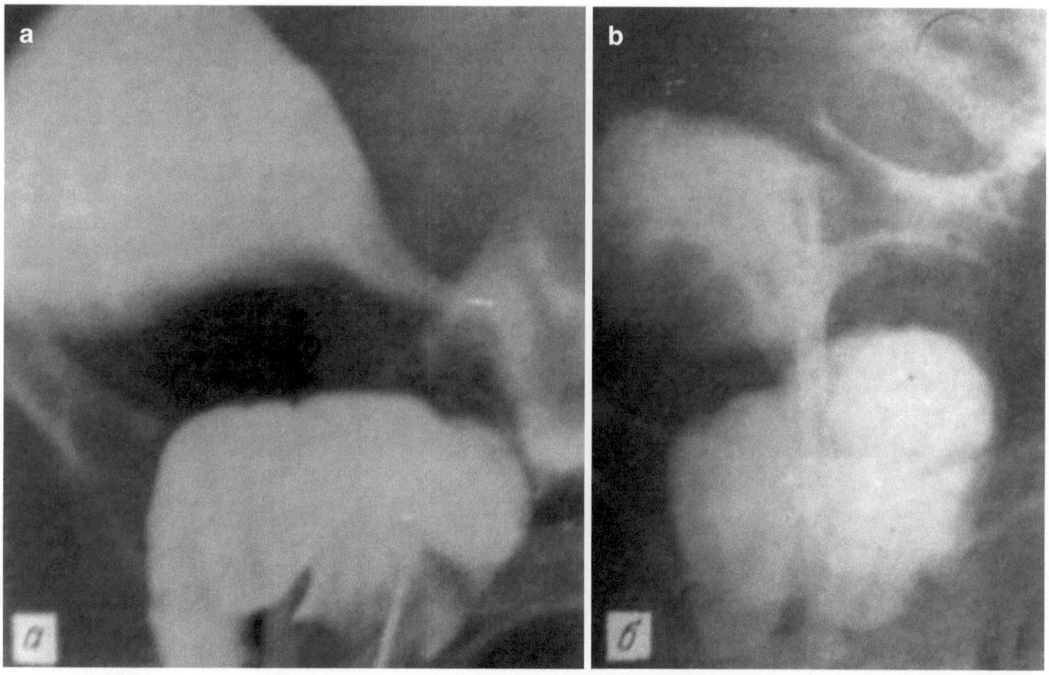

Fig. 4.11 (**a**) Puncture radiography of a cyst: the urinary bladder edged out to the right and upward with a multilocular formation at the level of the pubic articulation (the puncture needle was inserted transvaginally); (**b**) drainage of the urinary bladder through a rubber catheter inserted into the urethra that is surrounded by the paraurethral cysts in the shape of a horseshoe (After Terpigoriev and Builova [28])

of the paraurethral formation, its expansion, and connection with the surrounding tissues. These data are very important for defining the scope of the prospective surgical treatment (Figs. 4.12 and 4.13).

As noted by Pushkar and Anisimov [3], during MRI, apart from the paraurethral cyst/urethral diverticulum itself, ectatic paraurethral glands are visualized in some cases which is a condition for a repeated formation of the paraurethral cyst/UTHD (Figs. 4.11 and 4.12).

According to data provided by some authors [14], MRI allows classification of diverticula as simple, horseshoe-shaped, and round ones, in 10–57% cases of patients with DU. Although MRI facilitates understanding of the surgical anatomy of urethral diverticula, it does not possess any relevant clinical diagnostic value which is expressed only in one work by Pereverzev [18]; on the contrary, the majority of authors highly value the possibilities of MRI in UTHD diagnostics [3, 32, 38]. According to Verma and Mitchell [30]: "…MRI provides an excellent tissue contrasting and possibility of multiplane reconstructions which facilitates a detail study of the female urethra, anatomy and clarification of the lesion degree that is very beneficial for the surgery planning. Discharge from the urethra in case of UTHD is displayed like a vivid hyperintensive signal in the T2 weighted image near or around the urethra. Upon introduction of magnetic resonance contrast media which contain gadolinium no accumulation of gadolinium in UTHD is observed."

Nowadays thanks to the introduction of such noninvasive methods of ray diagnostics as USG and MRI, in the opinion of Pushkar and Anisimov [3], puncture of a discovered formation for diagnostical purposes, both for puncture radiography of a cyst and study of the contents, is no longer necessary. This is due to the fact that this manipulation is related with a high risk of infectious complications and also leads to complicated allocation of the cyst during the surgery.

When choosing an ray diagnostics algorithm for UTHD, noninvasive methods are currently preferable (Figs. 4.9 and 4.14).

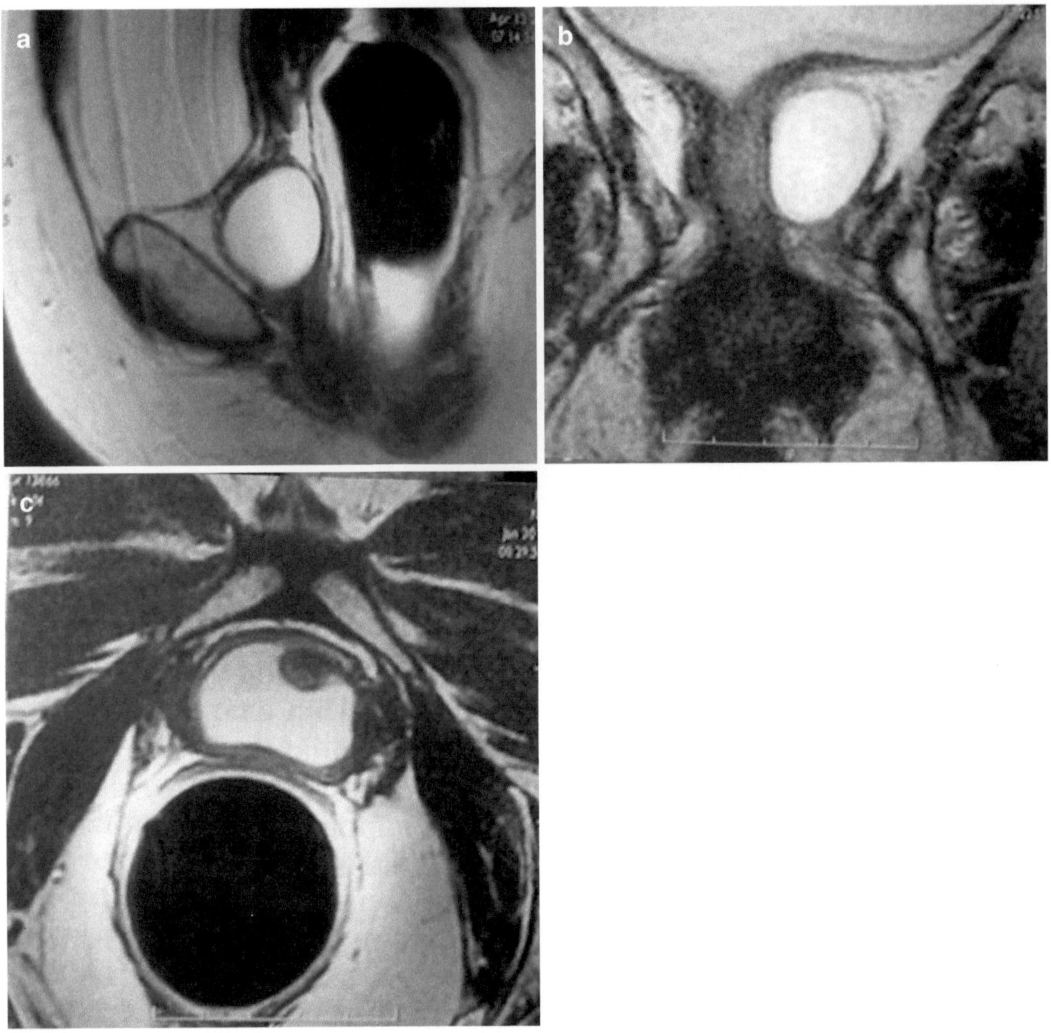

Fig. 4.12 Magnetic resonance images of the paraurethral cysts: (**a**) sagittal section; (**b**) frontal section; (**c**) axial section (After Pushkar and Anisimov [3])

As noted by Pushkar and Anisimov [3], during MRI, apart from the paraurethral cyst (urethral diverticulum) itself, ectatic paraurethral glands are visualized in some cases which is a condition for a repeated formation of the paraurethral cyst or UTHD (Figs. 4.11 and 4.12).

During recent years, upon introduction of modern multislice (detector) spiral computer tomographs (MSCT), in the urological clinic of the Sechenov Moscow Medical Academy, a *multidetector (multislice) spiral voiding cystourethrography* was developed [31, 32] which allowed to define not only the anatomical status of the urethra but also the depth of tissue affected by the pathological process and to perform the so-called virtual urethroscopy (Fig. 4.15). The relative disadvantages of this method are their high cost and rather a strong exposure of the patient's genital organs to radiation.

4.2.4 Differential Diagnostics

Although anamnesis and objective examination provide rather clear indications of UTHD, other nosologic units may be "disguised" as this

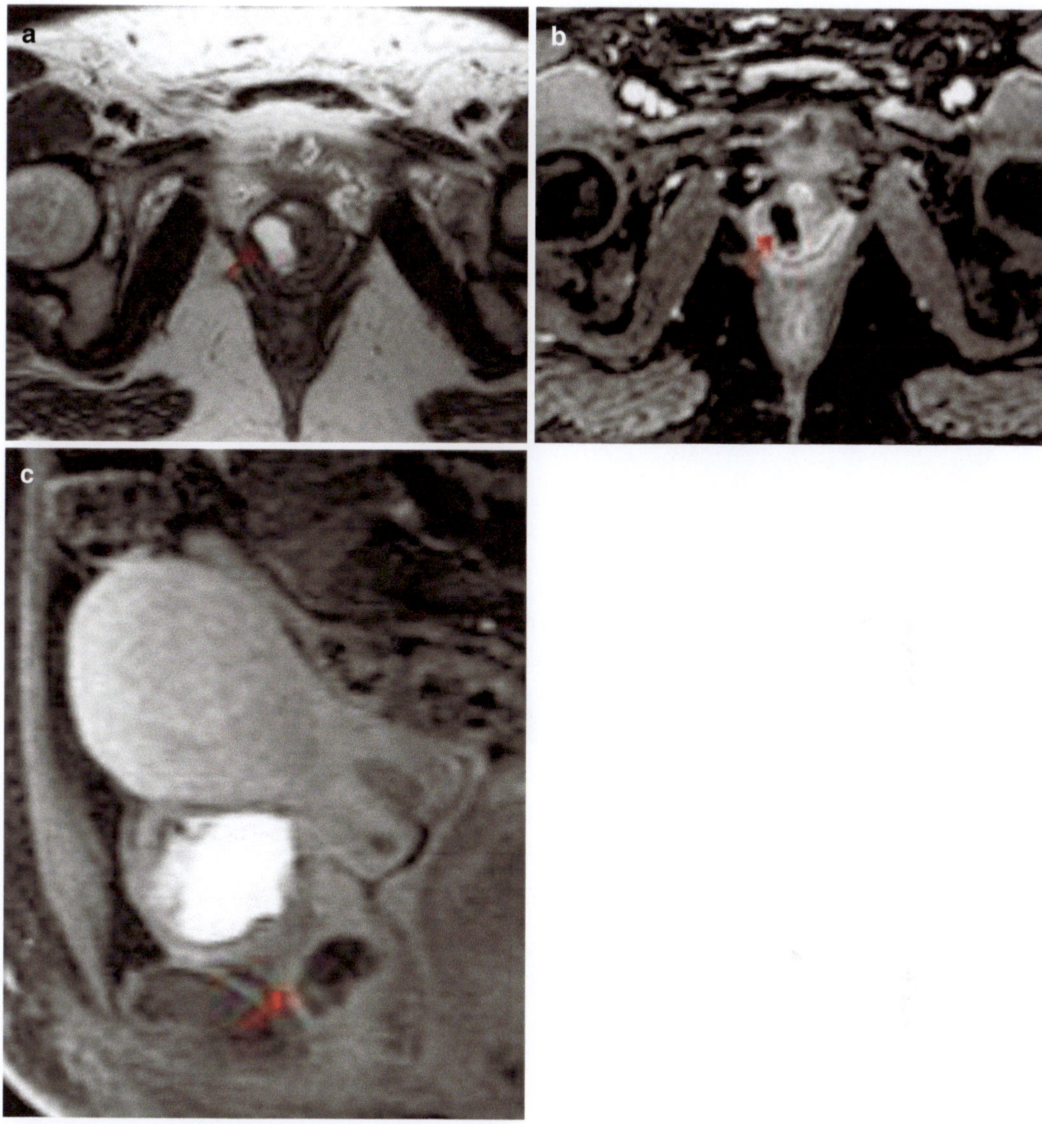

Fig. 4.13 (**a–c**) MRI of a 37-year-old woman with a recurrent urinary infection: (**a**) axial T2-weighted MR image of the pelvis displays a diverticular sac (*arrows*) near the right wall of the urethra which accumulates liquid; (**b**, **c**) axial and sagittal T1-weighted image prior to and after injection of a gadolinium containing MRCM does not display an increase in intensity of the diverticular sac (*arrow*) (Kim [38])

disease. A possibility of the simple bacterial cystitis must be kept in mind, and rather often painful feeling in the urinary bladder projection in combination with irritative symptoms accompanies the interstitial cystitis. Female urethra diverticulum can be imitated by a number of intravaginal and suburethral formations including abscesses of Skene glands that localize in the distal urethra without UTHD formation. Usually they are located to the side from the centerline. The misplaced ureter may reach the suburethral area. Presence of a misplaced ureter with a cystous dilatation and opening into the urethra can be excluded by means of an excretory urogram, voiding cystourethrograms, and cystourethroscopy. The most common pathological conditions of the female urethra which must be differentiated during diagnostics are ureterocele and

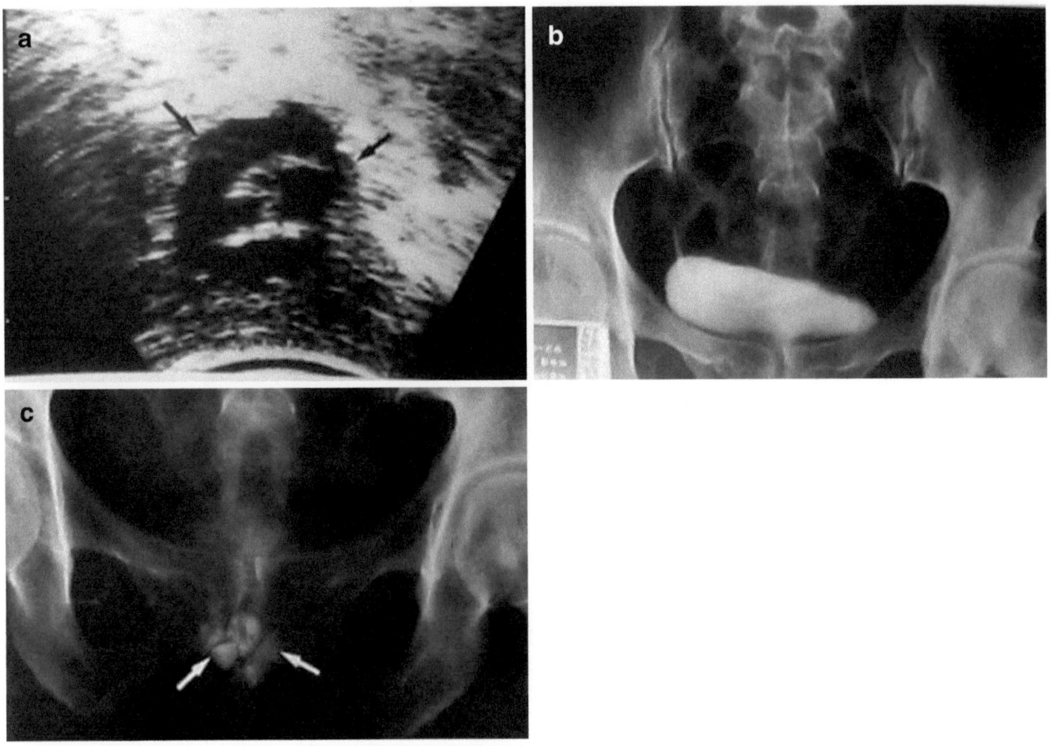

Fig. 4.14 (**a–c**) Urethral diverticulum of a 66-year-old female patient with recurrent cystitis: (**a**) a cystous formation with a thick septa (*arrows*) in the periurethral area visualized by means of transperineal USG; (**b**) the descending cystogram unchanged; (**c**) residual contrast medium (*arrows*) in a multilocular periurethral diverticulum in the image made after urination (Kim [38])

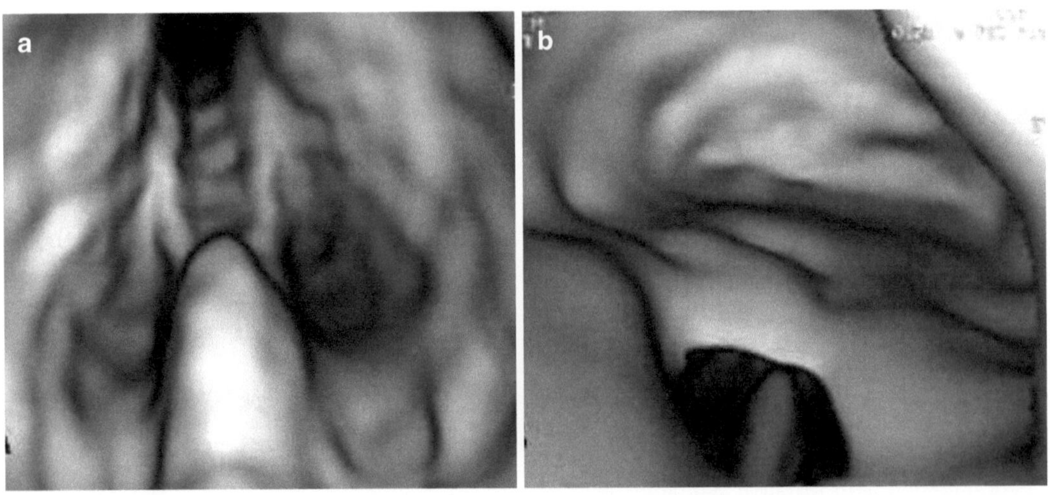

Fig. 4.15 Multidetector (multislice) spiral voiding cystourethrography: (**a, b**) virtual urethroscopy; (**c**) three-dimensional reconstruction; (**d, e**) voiding cystourethrograms in the frontal and sagittal projections (After Gazimiev and Builov [32])

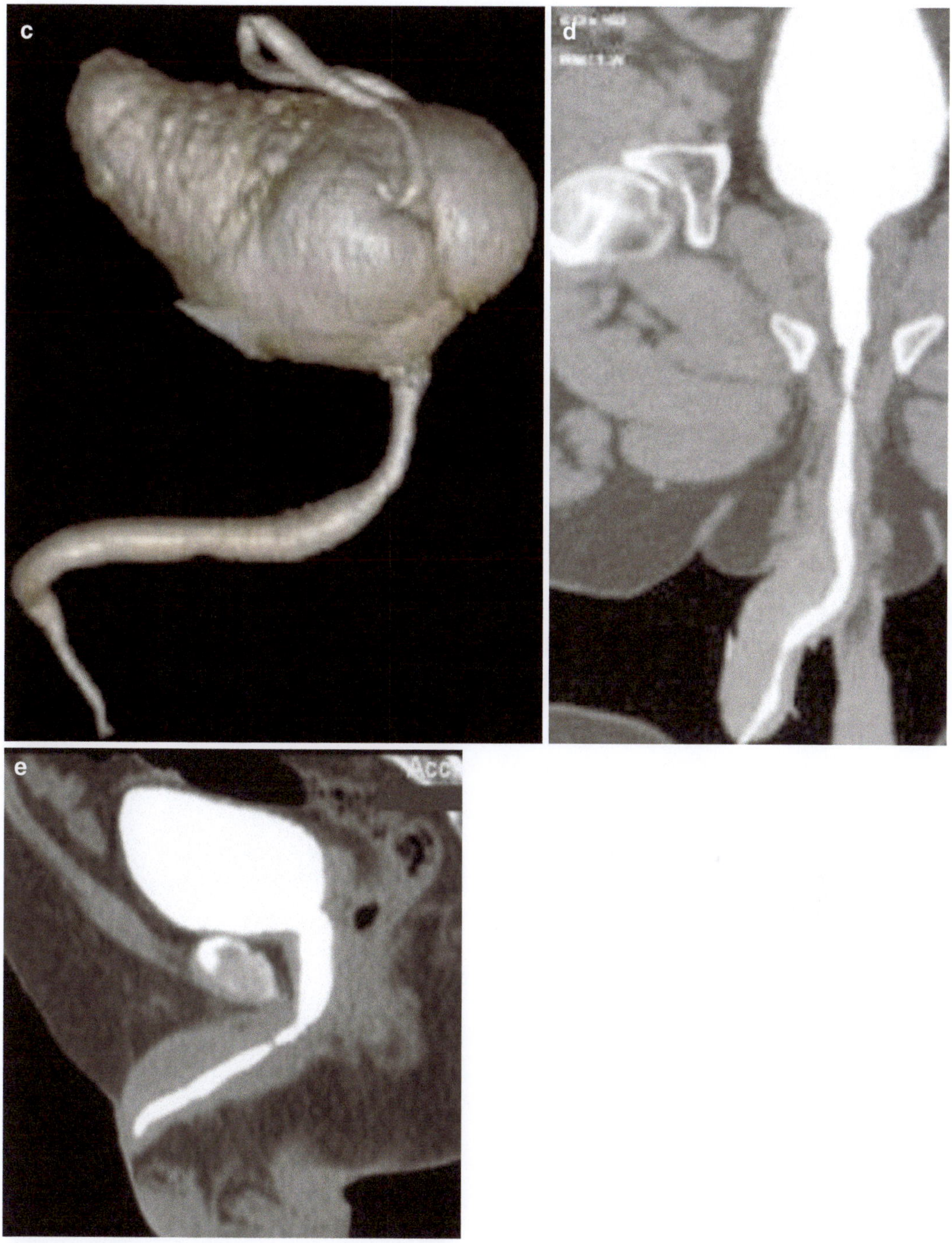

Fig. 4.15 (continued)

paraurethral cysts, a kind of "urine pockets," where urine or cyst contents accumulate. And, of course, urethra neoplasms may look like a suburethral palpable ecphyma.

The differential diagnosis must include all diseases manifested by suburethral tumorous formations. These are invasive transitional cell carcinoma, adenocarcinoma and squamous cell cancer, nephrogenic adenoma, and endometriosis. Paraurethral cysts do not have a visible communication with the urethra, but they are most probably remnants of diverticula with closed orifices.

4.3 Male Urethra Diverticula

UTHD is considered a rare disease in men. By 1924 Ilyin summarized 140 UTHD cases from the world literature (56, congenital; 84, acquired). The authors examined 109 patients after closed urethra injuries with fractures of pelvic bones and further surgical and conservative treatment; UTHD were discovered in 9 (8.2 %) patients. It is emphasized that timely surgery of infected UTHD prevents development of inflammatory diseases of the upper urinary tract [33–37]. Often the posttraumatic UTHD is complicated with lithogenesis, as well as with infection, which can also be self-developing [25, 33–37].

At the same time UTHD may not always be accompanied by the urethra blockade. Such a case was observed in a 16-year-old patient with UTHD which did not affect the UUT function and was an "accidental finding" [37]. USG and uroflowmetry in this patient displayed no deviation from the norm. No residual urine was detected. A complex urodynamic examination with profilometry confirmed a normal sensitivity and normotony of the urinary bladder. Signs of probably functional infravesical obstruction were discovered at the distance of 7.2–9.2 cm to the proximal side from the meatus. In order to clarify the state of the urethra, retrograde urethrography was performed where the urethra was visible all along its length and had the width of 0.6–1.1 cm. In the bulbar urethra, a cavity is visible, 2.5 × 1.5 cm, connected with the lumen with the end wide neck (Fig. 4.11). The prostatic urethra was displayed as a cavity up to 0.4 cm wide. With due consideration of reference data on possible disturbance of urination in patients with UTHD, an endoscopic dissection of the UTHD wall was performed (Fig. 4.12). However this treatment did not result in urination improvement. The effect was obtained after a course of drug therapy prescribed by a neurologist. Thus UTHD was not the cause of urination disturbance which turned out to be a result of the patient's psychological condition [37] (Figs. 4.16 and 4.17).

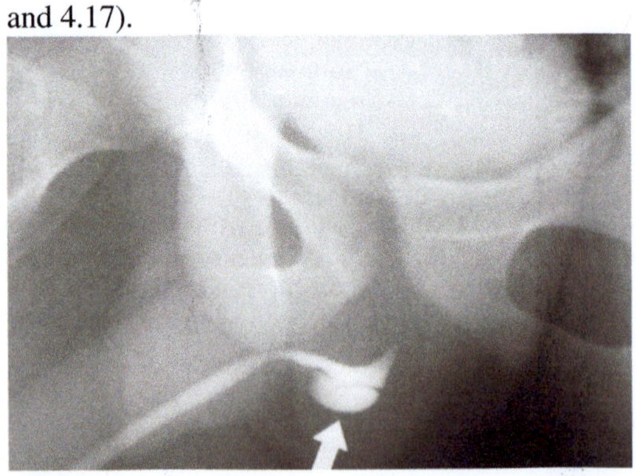

Fig. 4.16 Retrograde urethrography. The urethral diverticulum is shown with an *arrow* (After Rapoport et al. [37])

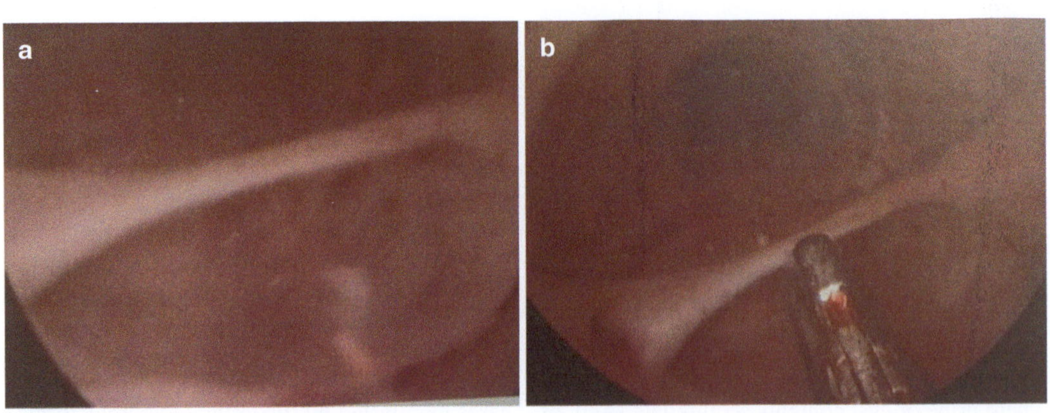

Fig. 4.17 Endophoto of the same patient: (**a**) urethroscopy, a pendant wall of the urethral diverticulum is visible; (**b**) dissection of the urethral diverticulum wall (After Rapoport et al. [37])

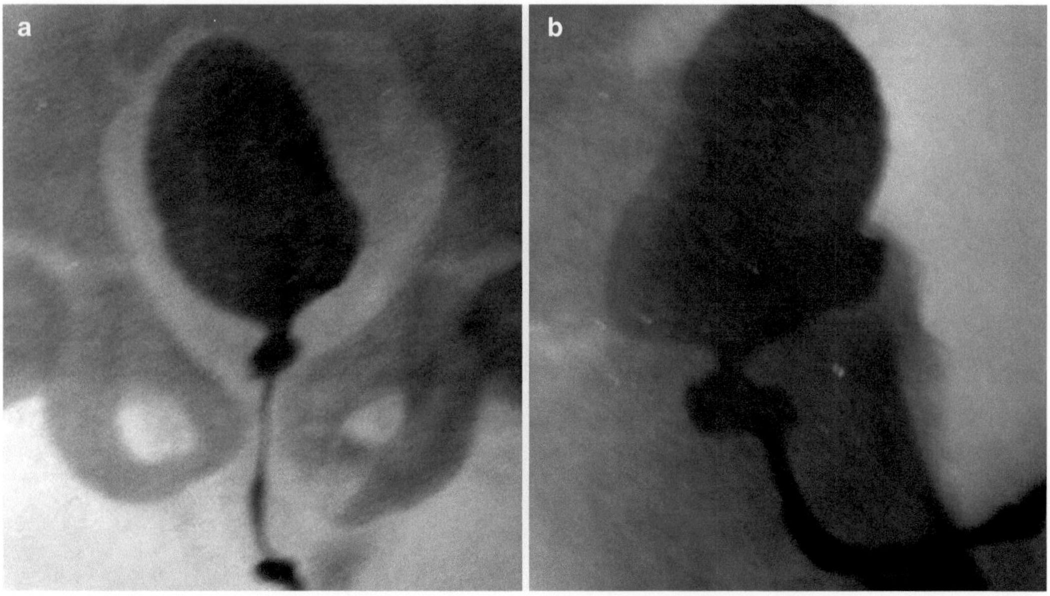

Fig. 4.18 (**a**, **b**) Ascending urethrocystograms in the front and oblique projections of a 5-year-old child with a congenital diverticulum of the rear urethra (After Tchukhrienko et al. [39])

Below is an example of rare localization of a congenital UTHD in the rear urethra of a 5-year-old boy (Fig. 4.18).

Unlike earlier cases, when discovered UTHD were obviously of the congenital nature and did not cause disturbance of urination, a development of an acquired diverticulum, especially of an iatrogenic character, with formation of a false duct (an urethral pseudodiverticulum) mostly produces the picture of urination disturbance due to urethra stricture (Figs. 4.19 and 4.20).

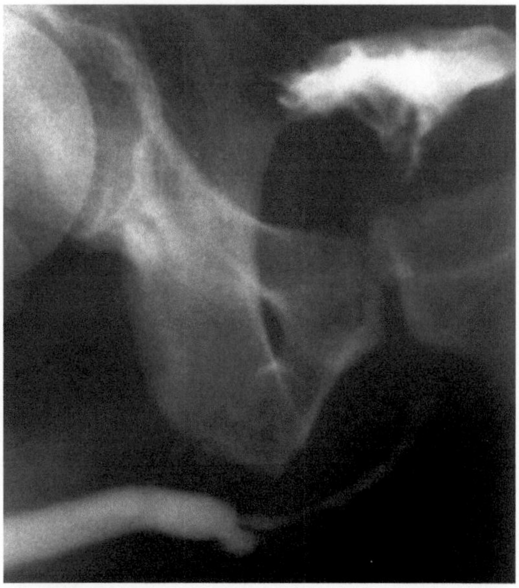

Fig. 4.19 Ascending urethrocystogram made under cineradiographic monitoring—filling of the urethral pseudodiverticulum ("a false duct" in the membranous urethra resulting from iatrogenic trauma after repetitive urethra bouginage); to the proximal side, a urethral stricture (*arrow*) about 0.1–0.2 cm long

4.3.1 Treatment

Treatment of UTHD requires surgical intervention which features nearly 20 % complication frequency rate. Surgery is justified for patients with prominent symptoms resulting from diverticulum presence. This includes recurrent urinary tract infections, pronounced pain, dyspareunia, polyuria, imperative feeling, and dribbling of urine after urination ("wet panties"), as well as such an accompanying condition as stress incontinence. There is no universal surgical method for treating patients with urethral diverticulum. If the diverticulum is very close to the external orifice of the urethra, it can be dissected through the urethra and vagina by means of marsupialization (Spence method). In rare cases endoscopic surgery by means of a urethroscope can be

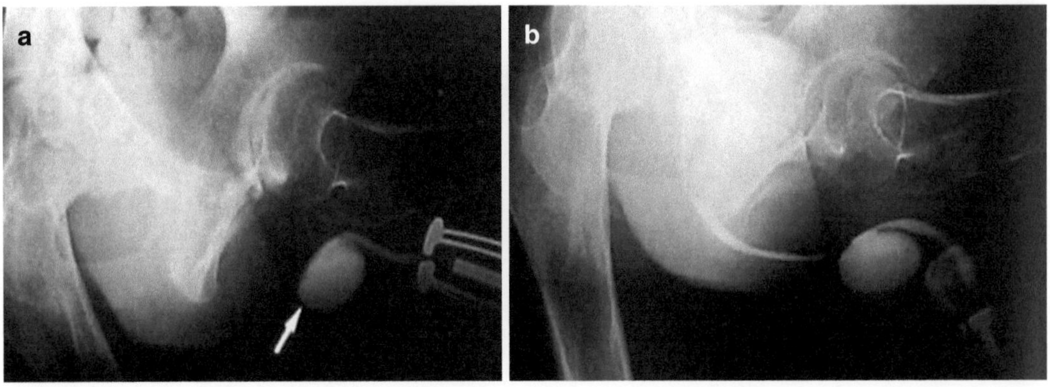

Fig. 4.20 (**a**, **b**) Diverticulum of the front urethra in a 22-year-old patient with paraplegia and prolonged urethral catheterization in anamnesis. (**a**) Retrograde urethrography reveals a large diverticulum (*arrow*) in the hanging part of the urethra near the penoscrotal segment. During further injection of the contrast medium, a diverticulum cavity is contrasted as well as its connection with the urethra. The patient complains of urine discharge upon pressing the "penile mass" (Kim [38])

performed. This will include electrocoagulation and expansion of the diverticulum orifice which will facilitate the diverticulum drainage.

A complete urethral diverticulectomy is the classical approach. Several methods are used; however the main idea consists in opening and mobilization of the diverticulum through a vaginal discission with the subsequent complete dissection of the diverticulum. The resulting small defect of the urethra is joined with fine stitch material. This method is a selection method due to possible discovery of a carcinoma in the diverticulum wall. According to [3], in spite of numerous proposed methods of conservative treatment for paraurethral cysts/UTHD, the treatment should be surgical and as radical as possible.

The removed cyst/diverticulum must be subject to histologic examination, since a transitional cell carcinoma may be discovered in situ in the UTHD wall, as well as adenocarcinoma, Paneth cell metaplasia, and endometriosis [5–10]. In these cases diverticulectomy is not a sufficient method of treatment.

4.4 Algorithms for UTHD Diagnostics

The leading methods of ray diagnostics of UTHD are X-ray methods with injection of a contrast medium in the ascending (retrograde) or descending, in case of EU, direction.

Among them the primary method is EU with descending voiding cystourethrography carried out under cineradiographic monitoring. Then in order to clarify the front urethra condition, men undergo ascending (retrograde) urethrography. Cineradiographic monitoring for controlling the degree of the urethra opacification during this process is mandatory. The direct monitoring of the XRCM injection via a display facilitates introduction of the optimum quantity to avoid the urethra hyperextension and development of unwanted XRCM extravasation.

It can be predicted that such modern methods as CAT and MRV, in course of decrease of their cost and improvement of availability, will be getting more and more common, along with USG and conventional ray diagnostics, in the area of X-ray UTHD diagnostics both in women and in men.

Finally it should be emphasized that UTHD, just as all other diverticula of the human organism in case of their congenital nature, generally do not produce any clinical presentations until complications develop. When this happens, it is time to move from observation and conservative treatment to making a decision concerning surgery. On the contrary, acquired UTHD have clinical presentations from the very beginning and require surgical correction. For all locations of diverticula in the upper and lower urinary tract, their advanced diagnostics is based on X-ray imaging methods.

References

1. Pytel AY, Pytel YA. X-ray diagnostics of urological diseases. Moscow: Meditsina; 1966. p. 385.
2. Mazhbits AM. Urogynecological surgery. Leningrad: Meditsina; 1964. p. 148.
3. Pushkar DY, Anisimov AV. Differential diagnostics and treatment of paraurethral cyst and/or urethral diverticulum. Urology. 2007;72(4):49–53.
4. Raz S. Female urology. 2nd ed. Philadelphia: W.B. Sanders Company; 1996. p. 477–89.
5. Zhorobekova AK. Paraurethral cysts in women. Thesis for the degree of Candidate of Medical Science, Philadelphia; 1992.
6. Hurt G. Urogynecologic surgery. Translation from the English language, editors Lopatkin NA, Apolikhin OI. Moscow: GEOTAR-MED; 2003. p. 221–33.
7. Blaivas JG, Flisser AJ, Bleustein CB, Panagopoulos G. Periurethral masses: etiology and diagnosis in a large series of women. Obstet Gynecol. 2004;103(5, pt 1): 842–7.
8. Clayton M, Siami P, Guinan P. Urethral diverticular carcinoma. Cancer. 1992;70(3):665–70.
9. Rajan N, Tucci P, Mallouh C. Carcinoma in female urethral diverticulum: case report and review of management. J Urol (Baltimore). 1993;150(6):1911–4.
10. Hruby G, Chao R, Lehman M, et al. Female clear cell adenocarcinoma arising within a urethral diverticulum. Can J Urol. 2000;7(6):1160–3.
11. Appell RA. Diverticulae of female uretrae. http//:www.Geicha.ru. Appell RA. Experience with a laterally based vaginal flap approach for urethral diverticulum. J Urol. 1982;127:677–8.
12. Appell RA. Urethral diverticulum and fistula. In: Glenn JF, editor. Urological surgery. 4th ed. Philadelphia: J. B. Lippincott; 1991. p. 762.
13. Drutz HP. Urethral diverticula. Obstet Gynecol Clin North Am. 1989;16:923–9.
14. Leech GE, Bavendam TG. Female urethral diverticula. Urology. 1987;40:407–15.
15. Leech GE, Sirls LT, Ganabathi K, Zimmern PE. LNSC3: a proposed classification system for female urethral diverticula. Neurourol Urodyn. 1993;12:523–31.
16. Spencer HM, Duckett JW. Diverticulum of the female urethra: clinical aspects and presentation of a single operative technique for care. J Urol. 1970;104:432–7.
17. Spencer WF, Streem SB. Diverticulum of the female urethral roof managed endoscopically. J Urol. 1987; 138:147–8.
18. Pereverzev AS. Female urethra diverticula. Medical aspects of female health. Edition for a practitioner. 2010;1(28):7–9.
19. Andersen MJ. The incidence of diverticula in the female urethra. J Urol. 1967;98:96–8.
20. Aspera AM, Rackley RR, Vasavada SP. Contemporary evaluation and management of the female urethral diverticulum. Urol Clin North Am. 2002;29:617–24.
21. Gomez-Lanza E. Female urethral diverticulum – a case report. Eur Urol Today. 2007;1:16.
22. Davis HJ, Telinde RW. Urethral diverticula: an assay of 121 cases. J Urol. 1958;80:34–9.
23. Davis BL, Robinson DG. Diverticula of the female urethra: assay of 120 cases. J Urol. 1970;104:850–3.
24. Hoffman JW. The detailed anatomy of the paraurethral ducts in the adult human female. Am J Obstet Gynecol. 1948;55:86–92.
25. Chowdhry AA, Miller FH, Hammer RA. Endometriosis presenting as a urethral diverticulum. A case report. J Reprod Med. 2004;49:321.
26. Romanzi LJ, Groutz A, Blaivas JG. Urethral diverticulum in women: diverse presentations resulting in diagnostic delay and mismanagement. J Urol. 2000;164:428.
27. Stepanov VN, Goldin YM. Cystous diseases of paraurethral glands in women. Urol Nephrol. 1974;(1):25–7.
28. Terpigoriev AM, Builova LA, Builov VM. Paraurethral cysts in women in practice of a dermatovenerologist. Dermatol Venereol Bull. 1987;(10):61–2.
29. Mukhtarov AM, Bolgarsky IS, Gajbullaev AV. On female urethra diverticula. Lib.: 8-th All-Russia Conference of Urologists. Abstracts of reports, 22–25 June 1988. Moscow; 1988. p. 79–80.
30. Verma SK, Mitchell DG. Female urethral diverticulum Posted Mon, 08/03/2009 18:22 by sverma Thomas Jefferson University Hospital, Philadelphia. http://imagingsciencetoday.com/teaching-case/gu-radiology/20090803/female-urethral-diverticulum-289.html.
31. Alyaev YG, Ternovoj SK, Grigoryan VA, et al. Voiding spiral tomography in diagnostics of urethral diseases. Urology. 2001;(5):23–6.
32. Gazimiev MA, Builov VM. Modern diagnostics of obstructive diseases in urology. Medical visualisation. Special edition. Materials of the 2nd All-Russia National Congress of Ray Diagnostics and Therapy. Moscow; 26–29 May 2008. p. 64–7.
33. Bolgarsky IS, Saidmuratov TD, Miroshnikov AV. Male urethra diverticulum. Lib.: diagnostics and treatment of male reproductive organs. Collection of scientific papers. Tashkent; 1987. p. 17–8.
34. Sachkov AF, Sergeev VA, Zajnutdinov RA. A case of acquired posttraumatic diverticulum in the distal urethra with formation of a giant stone. Lib.:: abstracts of the 13th Science and Practice Conference of Doctors of the Ulyanovsk Region dedicated to the 108th anniversary of V. I. Lenin, Ulyanovsk; 1978. p. 112–3.
35. Biryukov AA. Rear urethra diverticula in males after a trauma. Lib.: actual aspects of urology. Kemerovo; 1973. p. 165–6.
36. Dubensky VV. Persistent chlamydia infection in a patient with an urethral diverticulum. Russ Mag Dermatovenerol Dis. 2002;(1):50–3.
37. Rapoport L, Tsaritchenko D, Stojlov S, et al. Urethra diverticulum in a young patient. Doctor. 2007;(6):69–70.
38. Kim SH, editor. Radiology. Illustrated Uroradiology. Philadelphia: Saunders; 2003. p. 569.
39. Tchukhrienko AP, Lyulko AV, Lukich VA. Atlas of X-ray diagnostics of urological diseases. Moscow Meduchposobije; 1969. p. 123.
40. Talner LB, O'Reily PH, Wassereman NF. Specific causes of obstruction. In: Pollack HM, McClennan BL, editors. Clinical urography, vol. 2. 2nd ed. Philadelphia: WB Saunders; 2000. p. 1967–2136.

Appendix

Appendix 1: Guidelines of European Society of Urogenital Radiology (ESUR) on Contrast Media 8.1

ESUR Contrast Media Guidelines Version 8.1 (*Published with the permission of the Professor Henrik S. Thomsen, Chairman ESUR Contrast Media Safety Committee*)

Welcome to the ESUR Contrast Media Guidelines Version 8.1! We hope that you find our guidelines very helpful in your daily practice. We have modernized the layout to make it user-friendly as well as stylish. Due to the use of responsive templates, the web version can be viewed on any screen size, tablet, or even smartphones without the need for an additional application. The guidelines will successively be translated into many major languages—look out for yours! The Contrast Media Safety Committee has published 23 papers and books dealing with contrast media since its start in 1994. Please refer to "Publications" in the following web version. We hope you enjoy!

The Contrast Media Safety Committee of the European Society of Urogenital Radiology is proud to present the 8th version of its Contrast Media Guidelines. Version 7.0 was released 4 years ago and has been translated into Russian, Chinese, French, Italian, Spanish, Portuguese, Hungarian, German, Romanian, Polish, Greek, Japanese, Persian, Czech, and Turkish. Since our first guidelines were published, more than 100,000 copies have been printed. No other contrast medium guidelines have been printed in such numbers or so many languages. Our key aim of providing simple practical guidelines appears to have been fulfilled.

In Version 8.1, the guidelines on contrast medium-induced nephropathy, dialysis, late adverse reactions, and gadolinium-based contrast media and nephrogenic systemic fibrosis have been updated. The section on liver-specific agents has been omitted, because iron and manganese are no longer available in some countries and the issues regarding gadolinium-based liver-specific agents are covered in the section on extracellular gadolinium-based agents. We hope that you like the new booklet, that it is helpful in your practice, and that it will benefit all our patients. In 2013, the third edition of the book *Contrast Media: Safety Issues and ESUR Guidelines* (Springer, Germany) will be published. It provides the rationale for the guidelines in this booklet. Comments and questions are welcome at the ESUR webpage, www.esur.org, where these guidelines can be found in an electronic version.

ESUR Contrast Media Safety Committee May 2012

Henrik S. Thomsen, Chairman

In Version 8.1, section "Contrast Media and Catecholamine-Producing Tumors (Pheochromocytoma and Paraganglioma)" has been updated.

Nonrenal Adverse Reactions

Acute Adverse Reactions

Definition: An adverse reaction is defined as a reaction which occurs within 1 h of contrast medium injection.

V.M. Builov, *Imaging of Urinary Tract Diverticula*,
DOI 10.1007/978-3-319-05383-7, © Springer International Publishing Switzerland 2014

Classification

Mild
- Nausea, mild vomiting
- Urticaria
- Itching

Moderate
- Severe vomiting
- Marked urticaria
- Bronchospasm
- Facial/laryngeal edema
- Vasovagal attack

Severe
- Hypotensive shock
- Respiratory arrest
- Cardiac arrest
- Convulsion

Acute Adverse Reactions to Iodine-Based Contrast Media

Risk Factors for Acute Reactions

Patient Related

Patient with a history of:
- Previous moderate or severe acute reaction (see section "Classification" above) to an iodine-based contrast agent
- Asthma
- Allergy requiring medical treatment

Contrast Medium Related
- High-osmolality ionic contrast media

To Reduce the Risk of an Acute Reaction

For All Patients
- Use a nonionic contrast medium.
- Keep the patient in the radiology department for 30 min after contrast medium injection.
- Have the drugs and equipment for resuscitation readily available (see section "Management").

For Patients at Increased Risk of Reaction (See section "Risk Factors for Acute Reactions" Above)
- Consider an alternative test not requiring an iodine-based contrast agent.
- Use a different iodine-based agent for previous reactors to contrast medium.
- Consider the use of premedication. Clinical evidence of the effectiveness of premedication is limited. If used, a suitable premedication regime is prednisolone 30 mg (or methylprednisolone 32 mg), orally given 12 and 2 h before contrast medium.

Extravascular Administration of Iodine-Based Contrast Media
- When absorption or leakage into the circulation is possible, take the same precautions as for intravascular administration.

Acute Adverse Reactions to Gadolinium-Based Contrast Media

Note: The risk of an acute reaction to a gadolinium-based contrast agent is lower than the risk with an iodine-based contrast agent, but severe reactions to gadolinium-based contrast media may occur.

Risk Factors for Acute Reactions

Patient Related

Patient with a history of:
- Previous acute reaction to gadolinium-based contrast agent
- Asthma
- Allergy requiring medical treatment

Contrast Medium Related

The risk of reaction is not related to the osmolality of the contrast agent: The low doses used make the osmolar load very small.

To Reduce the Risk of an Acute Reaction

For All Patients
- Keep the patient in the radiology department for 30 min after contrast medium injection.
- Have the drugs and equipment for resuscitation readily available (see section "Management").

For Patients at Increased Risk of Reaction (See section "Risk Factors for Acute Reactions" Above)
- Consider an alternative test not requiring a gadolinium-based contrast agent.
- Use a different gadolinium-based agent for previous reactors to contrast medium.
- Consider the use of premedication. There is no clinical evidence of the effectiveness of premedication. If used, a suitable premedication regime is prednisolone 30 mg (or methylprednisolone 32 mg), orally given 12 and 2 h before contrast medium.

Management

First-line emergency drugs and instruments which should be in the examination room include:

Oxygen
Adrenaline 1:1,000
Atropine
β2-agonist metered dose inhaler
I.V. fluids—normal saline or Ringer's solution
Anticonvulsive drugs (diazepam)
Sphygmomanometer
One-way mouth "breather" apparatus

Simple Guidelines for First-Line Treatment of Acute Reactions to All Contrast Media

The same reactions are seen after iodine- and gadolinium-based contrast agents and after ultrasound contrast agents. The incidence is highest after iodine-based contrast agents and lowest after ultrasound agents.

Nausea/Vomiting

Transient: Supportive treatment.

Severe, protracted: Appropriate antiemetic drugs should be considered.

Urticaria

Scattered, transient: Supportive treatment including observation.

Scattered, protracted: Appropriate H1 antihistamine intramuscularly or intravenously should be considered. Drowsiness and/or hypotension may occur.

Generalized: Appropriate H1 antihistamine intramuscularly or intravenously should be given. Drowsiness and/or hypotension may occur. Consider adrenaline 1:1,000 0.1–0.3 ml (0.1–0.3 mg) intramuscularly in adults; 50 % of adult dose is to be given to pediatric patients between 6 and 12 years old, and 25 % of adult dose to pediatric patients below 6 years old, repeat as needed.

Bronchospasm

1. Oxygen by mask (6–10 l/min)
2. β2-agonist metered dose inhaler (2–3deepinhalations)
3. Adrenaline

Normal blood pressure

Intramuscular: 1:1,000 0.1–0.3 ml (0.1–0.3 mg) (use smaller dose in a patient with coronary artery disease or elderly patient)

In pediatric patients: 50 % of adult dose to pediatric patients between 6 and 12 years old and 25 % of adult dose to pediatric patients below 6 years old, repeat as needed

Decreased blood pressure

Intramuscular: 1:1,000 0.5 ml (0.5 mg)

In pediatric patients: 6–12 years—0.3 ml (0.3 mg) intramuscularly

<6 years—0.15 ml (0.15 mg) intramuscularly

Laryngeal Edema

1. Oxygen by mask (6–10 l/min)
2. Intramuscular adrenaline 1:1,000 0.5 ml (0.5 mg) for adults, repeat as needed
   In pediatric patients: 6–12 years—0.3 ml (0.3 mg) intramuscularly
   <6 years—0.15 ml (0.15 mg) intramuscularly

Hypotension

Isolated hypotension

1. Elevate patient's legs.
2. Oxygen by mask (6–10 l/min).
3. Intravenous fluid: rapidly, normal saline or Ringer's solution.
4. If unresponsive: adrenaline 1:1,000 0.5 ml (0.5 mg) intramuscularly, repeat as needed
   In pediatric patients: 6–12 years—0.3 ml (0.3 mg) intramuscularly
   <6 years—0.15 ml (0.15 mg) intramuscularly

Vagal reaction (hypotension and bradycardia)

1. Elevate patient's legs.
2. Oxygen by mask (6–10 l/min).
3. Atropine 0.6–1.0 mg intravenously, repeat if necessary after 3–5 min, to 3 mg total (0.04 mg/kg) in adults. In pediatric patients give 0.02 mg/kg intravenously (max. 0.6 mg per dose), repeat if necessary to 2 mg total.
4. Intravenous fluids: rapidly, normal saline or Ringer's solution.

Generalized Anaphylactoid Reaction

1. Call for resuscitation team.
2. Suction airway as needed.
3. Elevate patient's legs if hypotensive.
4. Oxygen by mask (6–10 l/min)
5. Intramuscular adrenaline (1:1,000), 0.5 ml (0.5 mg) in adults, repeat as needed
   In pediatric patients: 6–12 years—0.3 ml (0.3 mg) intramuscularly
   <6 years—0.15 ml (0.15 mg) intramuscularly

6. Intravenous fluids (e.g., normal saline, Ringer's solution).
7. H1-blocker, e.g., diphenhydramine 25–50 mg intravenously.

Late Adverse Reactions

Definition: A late adverse reaction to intravascular iodine-based contrast medium is defined as a reaction which occurs 1 h to 1 week after contrast medium injection.

Reactions

Skin reactions are similar in type to other drug-induced eruptions. Maculopapular rashes, erythema, swelling, and pruritus are the most common. Most skin reactions are mild to moderate and self-limiting.

A variety of late symptoms (e.g., nausea, vomiting, headache, musculoskeletal pains, fever) have been described following contrast medium, but many are not related to contrast medium.

Risk Factors for Skin Reactions

- Previous late contrast medium reaction
- Interleukin-2 treatment
- Use of nonionic dimers

Management

Symptomatic and similar to the management of other drug-induced skin reactions, e.g., antihistamines, topical steroids, and emollients

Recommendations

Patients who have had a previous contrast medium reaction or who are on interleukin-2 treatment should be advised that a late skin reaction is possible and that they should contact a doctor if they have a problem.

Patch and delayed-reading intradermal tests may be useful to confirm a late skin reaction to contrast medium and to study cross-reactivity patterns with other agents.

To reduce the risk of repeat reaction, use another contrast agent than the agent precipitating the first reaction. Avoid agents which have shown cross-reactivity on skin testing.

Drug prophylaxis is generally not recommended.

Note: Late skin reactions of the type which occur after iodine-based contrast media have not been described after gadolinium-based and ultrasound contrast media.

Very Late Adverse Reactions

Definition: An adverse reaction is a reaction which usually occurs more than 1 week after contrast medium injection.

Types of Reaction

Iodine-based contrast media: thyrotoxicosis

Gadolinium-based contrast media: nephrogenic systemic fibrosis

Thyrotoxicosis

At Risk

- Patients with untreated Graves' disease
- Patients with multinodular goiter and thyroid autonomy, especially if they are elderly and/or live in area of dietary iodine deficiency

Not at Risk

- Patients with normal thyroid function

Recommendations

- *Iodinated contrast media should not be given to patients with manifest hyperthyroidism.*
- Prophylaxis is generally not necessary.
- In selected high-risk patients, prophylactic treatment may be given by an endocrinologist; this is more relevant in areas of dietary iodine deficiency.
- Patients at risk should be closely monitored by endocrinologists after iodine- based contrast medium injection.
- Intravenous cholangiographic contrast media should not be given to patients at risk.

Nephrogenic Systemic Fibrosis

A diagnosis of nephrogenic systemic fibrosis (NSF) should only be made if the Yale NSF Registry clinical and histopathological criteria are met (*J Am Acad Dermatol* 2011;65:1095–106). The link between nephrogenic systemic fibrosis (NSF) and gadolinium-based contrast agents was recognized in 2006.

Clinical Features of NSF

Onset: From the day of exposure for up to 2–3 months, sometimes up to years after exposure

Initially

- Pain
- Pruritus
- Swelling

- Erythema
- Usually starts in the legs

Later

- Thickened skin and subcutaneous tissues—"woody" texture and brawny plaques
- Fibrosis of internal organs, e.g., muscle, diaphragm, heart, liver, and lungs

Result

- Contractures
- Cachexia
- Death, in a proportion of patients

Patients at Higher Risk

- Patients with CKD 4 and 5 (GFR < 30 ml/min)
- Patients on dialysis
- Patients with acute kidney insufficiency

Patients at Lower Risk

- Patients with CKD 3 (GFR 30–59 ml/min)
- Patients Not at Risk
- Patients with stable GFR > 60 ml/min

Contrast Agents

Risk Classification (Based on Laboratory Data) and Recommendations

Highest Risk of NSF

Contrast Agents

Gadodiamide (Omniscan®)

- Ligand: nonionic linear chelate (DTPA-BMA)
- Incidence of NSF: 3–18 % in at-risk subjects

Gadopentetate dimeglumine (Magnevist® plus generic products)

- Ligand: ionic linear chelate (DTPA)
- Incidence of NSF: estimated to be 0.1–1 % in at-risk subjects

Gadoversetamide (Optimark®)

- Ligand: nonionic linear chelate (DTPA-BMEA)
- Incidence of NSF: unknown

Recommendations

These agents are CONTRAINDICATED in:

- Patients with CKD 4 and 5 (GFR < 30 ml/min), including those on dialysis
- Patients with acute renal insufficiency
- Pregnant women
- Neonates

These agents should be used with CAUTION in:

- Patients with CKD 3 (GFR 30–60 ml/min): There should be at least 7 days between two injections.
- Children less than 1 year old.

Lactating women: Stop breastfeeding for 24 h and discard the milk.

Serum creatinine (eGFR) measurement and clinical assessment of patient before administration is *mandatory*.

These agents should never be given in doses higher than 0.1 mmol/kg per examination in any patient.

Intermediate Risk of NSF

Contrast Agents

Gadobenate dimeglumine (MultiHance®)

- Ligand: ionic linear chelate (BOPTA).
- Incidence of NSF: No unconfounded* cases have been reported.
- Special feature: It is a combined extracellular and liver-specific agent with 2–3 % albumin binding. Diagnostic results can be achieved with 50 % lower doses than with the usual extracellular agents. In man ~4 % is excreted via the liver.

Gadofosveset trisodium (Vasovist®, Ablavar®)

- Ligand: ionic linear chelate (DTPA-DPCP).
- Incidence of NSF: No unconfounded* cases reported, but experience is limited.
- Special feature: It is a blood pool agent with affinity to albumin (>90 %). Diagnostic results can be achieved with 50 % lower doses than extracellular Gd-CM. Biological half-life is 12 times longer than for extracellular agents (18 h compared to 11⁄2 h, respectively); 5 % is excreted via the bile.

Gadoxetate disodium (Primovist®, Eovist®)

- Ligand: ionic linear chelate (EOB-DTPA)
- Incidence of NSF: No unconfounded* cases have been reported but experience is limited.
- Special feature: It is an organ-specific gadolinium contrast agent with 10 % protein binding and 50 % excretion by hepatocytes. Diagnostic results can be achieved with lower doses than extracellular Gd-CM.

Recommendations

These agents should be used with CAUTION in:

- Patients with CKD 4 and 5 (GFR < 30 ml/min): There should be at least 7 days between two injections.

Pregnant women: can be used to give essential diagnostic information.

Lactating women: The patient should discuss with the doctor whether the breast milk should be discarded in the 24 h after contrast medium injection.

Laboratory testing of renal function (eGFR) is *not mandatory*. Renal function assessment by questionnaire should be used if serum creatinine is not measured.

Lowest Risk of NSF

Contrast Agents

Gadobutrol (Gadovist®, Gadavist®)

- Ligand: nonionic cyclic chelate (BT-DO3A).
- Incidence of NSF: A few unconfounded* cases have been reported, but there is uncertainty about the histopathological changes.

Gadoterate meglumine (Dotarem®, Magnescope®)

- Ligand: ionic cyclic chelate (DOTA).
- Incidence of NSF: No unconfounded* cases have been reported.

Gadoteridol (ProHance®)

- Ligand: nonionic cyclic chelate (HP-DO3A).
- Incidence of NSF: No unconfounded* cases have been reported.

Recommendations

These agents should be used with CAUTION in:

- Patients with CKD 4 and 5 (GFR < 30 ml/min): There should be at least 7 days between two injections.

Pregnant women: can be used to give essential diagnostic information.

Lactating women: The patient should discuss with the doctor whether the breast milk should be discarded in the 24 h after contrast medium injection.

Laboratory testing of renal function (eGFR) is *not mandatory*. Renal function assessment by questionnaire should be used if serum creatinine is not measured.

Patients with NSF

Gadolinium-based contrast media should only be used if the indication is vital, and then only intermediate- or low-risk agents should be used.

Recommendation for All Patients

Never deny a patient a clinically well- indicated enhanced MRI examination. In all patients use the smallest amount of contrast medium necessary for a diagnostic result.

Always record the name and dose of the contrast agent used in the patient records.

**Confounded cases*: If two different Gd-CM have been injected, it is impossible to determine with certainty which agent triggered the development of NSF, and the situation is described as "confounded."

Unconfounded cases: The patient has never been exposed to more than one agent.

Renal Adverse Reactions

Definition: Contrast medium-induced nephropathy (CIN) is a condition in which a decrease in renal function occurs within 3 days of the intravascular administration of a CM in the absence of an alternative etiology. An increase in serum creatinine by more than 25 % or 44 μmol/l (0.5 mg/dl) indicates CIN.

Renal Adverse Reactions to Iodine-Based Contrast Media

Risk Factors for Contrast Medium-Induced Nephropathy

Patient Related

- eGFR less than 60 ml/min/1.73 m^2 before intra-arterial administration
- eGFR less than 45 ml/min/1.73 m^2 before intravenous administration
- Diabetic nephropathy
- Dehydration
- Congestive heart failure (NYHA grade 3–4) and low LVEF
- Recent myocardial infarction (<24 h)
- Intra-aortic balloon pump
- Periprocedural hypotension
- Low hematocrit level
- Age over 70
- Concurrent administration of nephrotoxic drugs
- Known or suspected acute renal failure

Procedure Related

- Intra-arterial administration of contrast medium
- High-osmolality agents
- Large doses of contrast medium
- Multiple contrast medium administrations within a few days

Time of Referral

Elective Examination

Identify patients who require measurement of renal function.

Determine eGFR (or SCr) within 7 days of contrast medium administration:

- Patients with known eGFR less than 60 ml/min/1.73 m^2
- Patients who will receive intra-arterial contrast medium
- Patients aged over 70
- Patients with a history of:
  - Renal disease
  - Renal surgery
  - Proteinuria
  - Diabetes mellitus
  - Hypertension
  - Gout
  - Taking recent nephrotoxic drugs

Emergency Examination

- Identify at-risk patients (see above) if possible.
- Determine eGFR if the procedure can be deferred until the result is available without harm to the patient.
- If eGFR cannot be obtained, follow the protocols for patients with eGFR less than 60 ml/min/1.73 m^2 for intra-arterial administration and eGFR less than 45 ml/min/1.73 m^2 for intravenous administration as closely as clinical circumstances permit.

Before the Examination

Elective Examination

At-Risk Patients (See Above)

- Consider an alternative imaging method not using iodine-based contrast media.
- Discuss the need to stop nephrotoxic drugs with the referring physician.
- Start volume expansion. A suitable protocol is intravenous normal saline, 1.0–1.5 ml/kg/h, for at least 6 h before and after contrast medium injection. An alternative protocol is intravenous sodium bicarbonate (154 mEq/l in dextrose 5 % water), 3 ml/kg/h for 1 h before contrast medium injection and 1 ml/kg/h for 6 h after contrast medium injection.

Emergency Examination

At-Risk Patients (See Above)

- Consider an alternative imaging method not using iodine-based contrast media.
- Start volume expansion as early as possible before contrast medium administration (see section "Elective Examination").

Time of Examination

At-Risk Patients (See Above)

- Use low or isoosmolar contrast media.
- Use the lowest dose of contrast medium consistent with a diagnostic result.

Patients Not at Increased Risk

- Use the lowest dose of contrast medium consistent with a diagnostic result.

After the Examination

At-Risk Patients

- Continue volume expansion.
- Determine eGFR 48–72 h after contrast medium injection.

Note: No pharmacological prophylaxis (with renal vasodilators, receptor antagonists of endogenous vasoactive mediators, or cytoprotective drugs) has yet been shown to offer consistent protection against contrast medium-induced nephropathy.

Renal Adverse Reactions to Gadolinium-Based Contrast Media

MRI Examinations

- The risk of nephrotoxicity is very low when gadolinium-based contrast media are used in approved doses.
- In patients with reduced renal function, refer to ESUR guidelines on NSF (section "Nephrogenic Systemic Fibrosis").

Radiographic Examinations

- Gadolinium-based contrast media should not be used for radiographic examinations in patients with renal impairment.
- Gadolinium-based contrast media are more nephrotoxic than iodine-based contrast media in equivalent X-ray attenuating doses.

Patients Taking Metformin

Iodine-Based Contrast Media

1. Patients with eGFR equal to or greater than 60 ml/min/1.73 m^2 (CKD 1 and 2) can continue to take metformin normally.
2. Patients with eGFR 30–59 ml/min/1.73 m^2 (CKD 3):
   (a) Patients receiving intravenous contrast medium with eGFR equal to or greater than 45 ml/min/1.73 m^2 can continue to take metformin normally.
   (b) Patients receiving intra-arterial contrast medium and those receiving intravenous contrast medium with an eGFR between 30 and 44 ml/min/1.73 m^2 should stop metformin 48 h before contrast medium and should only restart metformin 48 h after contrast medium injection if renal function has not deteriorated.
3. Patients with eGFR less than 30 ml/min/1.73 m^2 (CKD 4 and 5) or with an intercurrent illness causing reduced liver function or hypoxia. Metformin is contraindicated and iodine-based contrast media should be avoided.
4. Emergency patients. Metformin should be stopped from the time of contrast medium administration. After the procedure, the patient should be monitored for signs of lactic acidosis. Metformin should be restarted 48 h after contrast medium injection if serum creatinine/eGFR is unchanged from the pre-imaging level.

Gadolinium-Based Contrast Media

No special precautions are necessary when diabetic patients on metformin are given gadolinium-based contrast medium.

Dialysis and Contrast Medium Administration

All iodine- and gadolinium-based contrast media can be removed by hemodialysis or peritoneal dialysis. However, there is no evidence that hemodialysis protects patients with impaired renal function from contrast medium-induced nephropathy or nephrogenic systemic fibrosis. In all patients, avoid osmotic and fluid overload. To avoid the risk of NSF, refer to section "Nephrogenic Systemic Fibrosis".

Patients on Dialysis

Hemodialysis

Iodine-Based Contrast Medium

- Correlation of time of the contrast medium injection with the hemodialysis session is unnecessary.
- Extra hemodialysis session to remove contrast medium is unnecessary.

Gadolinium-Based Contrast Medium

- Correlation of time of the contrast medium injection with the hemodialysis session is recommended.
- Extra hemodialysis session to remove contrast medium as soon as possible after it has been administered is recommended.

Continuous Ambulatory Peritoneal Dialysis

Iodine-Based Contrast Medium

- Hemodialysis to remove the contrast medium is unnecessary for iodine-based contrast medium but necessary for gadolinium-based contrast medium. It should be discussed with the referring physician.

Gadolinium-Based Contrast Medium

- Hemodialysis to remove the contrast medium is unnecessary for iodine-based contrast medium but necessary for gadolinium- based contrast medium. It should be discussed with referring physician.

Miscellaneous

Contrast Medium Extravasation

Type of Injuries

- Most injuries are minor.
- Severe injuries include skin ulceration, soft tissue necrosis, and compartment syndrome.

Risk Factors Technique Related

- Use of a power injector
- Less optimal injection sites including lower limb and small distal veins

- Large volume of contrast medium
- High-osmolar contrast media

Patient Related

- Inability to communicate
- Fragile or damaged veins
- Arterial insufficiency
- Compromised lymphatic and/or venous drainage
- Obesity

To Reduce the Risk

- Intravenous technique should always be meticulous using appropriate-sized plastic cannula placed in a suitable vein to handle the flow rate used during the injection.
- Test injection with normal saline.
- Use nonionic iodine-based contrast medium.

Treatment

- Conservative management is adequate in most cases:
  Limb elevation
  Ice pack application
  Careful monitoring
- If a serious injury is suspected, seek the advice of a surgeon.

Pulmonary Effects of Iodine-Based Contrast Media

Pulmonary Adverse Effects

- Bronchospasm
- Increased pulmonary vascular resistance
- Pulmonary edema

Patients at High Risk

- History of asthma
- History of pulmonary hypertension
- Incipient cardiac failure

To Reduce the Risk of Pulmonary Adverse Effects

- Use low or isoosmolar contrast media.
- Avoid large doses of contrast media.

Effects of Iodine-Based Contrast Media on Blood and Endothelium

The clinically important adverse effect of iodine-based contrast media on blood and endothelium is thrombosis.

It is recognized that:

- All contrast media have anticoagulant properties, especially ionic agents.
- High-osmolar ionic contrast media may induce thrombosis due to endothelial damage, particularly in phlebographic procedures.
- Drugs and interventional devices that decrease the risk of thromboembolic complications during interventional procedures minimize the importance of the effects of contrast media.

Guidelines

- Meticulous angiographic technique is mandatory and is the most important factor in reducing thromboembolic complications.
- Low- or isoosmolar contrast media should be used for diagnostic and interventional angiographic procedures including phlebography.

Contrast Media and Catecholamine-Producing Tumors (Pheochromocytoma and Paraganglioma)

Preparation

(a) Before intravenous iodine- or gadolinium-based contrast medium: No special preparation is required.

(b) Before intra-arterial iodine-based contrast medium: α- and β-adrenergic blockade with orally administered drugs under the supervision of the referring physician is recommended.

Types of Contrast Medium Which Should Be Used

Iodine based: nonionic agent

Gadolinium based: any agent, ionic or nonionic

Pregnancy and Lactation

Pregnancy

(a) In exceptional circumstances, when radiographic examination is essential, iodine-based contrast media may be given to the pregnant female.

(b) Following administration of iodine-based agents to the mother during pregnancy, thyroid function should be checked in the neonate during the first week.

(c) When there is a very strong indication for enhanced MR, the smallest possible dose of one of the most stable gadolinium contrast agents (see Contrast Agents: Intermediate and Low Risk of NSF, section "Nephrogenic Systemic Fibrosis") may be given to the pregnant female.

(d) Following administration of gadolinium-based agents to the mother during pregnancy, no neonatal tests are necessary.

Lactation

- Breastfeeding may be continued normally when iodine-based agents are given to the mother.

- Breastfeeding should be avoided for 24 h after contrast medium injection if high-risk agents are used.

Pregnant or Lactating Mother with Renal Impairment

- See section "Renal Adverse Reactions" (see section "Renal Adverse Reactions to Iodine-Based Contrast Media"). No additional precautions are necessary for the fetus or neonate.
- Do not administer gadolinium-based contrast agents.

Interaction with Other Drugs and Clinical Tests

General Recommendation

- Be aware of the patient's drug history.
- Keep a proper record of the contrast medium injection (time, dose, name).
- Do not mix contrast media with other drugs in tubes and syringes.

Drugs Needing Special Attention

Metformin

Refer to renal adverse reactions (section "Renal Adverse Reactions to Iodine-Based Contrast Media").

Nephrotoxic Drugs

Cyclosporine

Cisplatin

Aminoglycosides

Nonsteroidal anti-inflammatory drugs

Refer to renal adverse reactions (section "Renal Adverse Reactions to Iodine-Based Contrast Media").

Beta-Blocker

β-blockers may impair the management of bronchospasm and the response to adrenaline.

Interleukin-2

Refer to late adverse reactions (section "Late Adverse Reactions").

Biochemical Assays

Recommendation

Do not perform nonemergency biochemical analysis of blood and urine collected in the 24 h after contrast medium injection.

Isotope Studies and/or Treatment

Thyroid

Patients undergoing therapy with radioactive iodine should not have received iodine-based contrast media for at least 2 months before treatment.

Isotope imaging of the thyroid should be avoided for 2 months after iodine-based contrast medium injection.

Bone, Red Blood Cell Labeling

Avoid iodine-based contrast medium injection for at least 24 h before the isotope study.

Safety of Ultrasound Contrast Media

Statement: Ultrasound contrast media are generally safe.

Contraindication: Severe heart disease (e.g., New York class III/IV)

Type and Severity of Reactions

- The majority of reactions are minor (e.g., headache, nausea, sensation of heat, altered taste) and self-resolving.
- More severe acute reactions are rare and are similar to those after iodine- and gadolinium-based agents (see section "Acute Adverse Reactions").

To Reduce the Risk

- Check for intolerance to any of the components of the contrast agent.
- Use the lowest level of acoustic output and shortest scanning time to allow a diagnostic examination.

Treatment: If a serious event occurs, see section "Nonrenal Adverse Reactions".

Safety of Barium Contrast Media

Contraindications

Contraindications

- Integrity of gut wall compromised
- Use iodine-based water-soluble contrast media
- In neonates and patients at risk of leakage into the mediastinum and/or lungs, use low- or isoosmolar contrast media.
- Previous allergic reactions to barium products
- Use iodine-based water-soluble contrast media and be prepared to treat a reaction.

Cautions
- Bowel strictures
- Use only small amounts.
- Extensive colitis
- Avoid barium enemas.

Complications
- Reduced bowel motility
- Encourage fluid intake.
- Venous intravasation
- Early identification and careful observation.
- Antibiotics and intravenous fluids.
- Emergency treatment may be needed.

Aspiration
- Bronchoscopic removal for large amounts
- Chest physiotherapy
- Antibiotics

Questionnaires

Questionnaires to be completed by clinicians referring patients for examinations using iodine- or gadolinium-based contrast media

Questionnaire for iodine-based contrast media administration to be completed by the referring clinician

1. History of moderate or severe reaction to an iodine-based contrast medium	☐ Yes ☐ No
2. History of allergy requiring treatment	☐ Yes ☐ No
3. History of asthma	☐ Yes ☐ No
4. Hyperthyroidism	☐ Yes ☐ No
5. Heart failure	☐ Yes ☐ No
6. Diabetes mellitus	☐ Yes ☐ No
7. History of renal disease	☐ Yes ☐ No
8. Previous renal surgery	☐ Yes ☐ No
9. History of proteinuria	☐ Yes ☐ No
10. Hypertension	☐ Yes ☐ No
11. Gout	☐ Yes ☐ No
12. Most recent measurement of serum creatinine	
Value	
Date	
13. Is the patient currently taking any of the following drugs:	
Metformin	☐ Yes ☐ No
Interleukin 2	☐ Yes ☐ No
NSAIDs	☐ Yes ☐ No
Aminoglycosides	☐ Yes ☐ No
☐-blockers	☐ Yes ☐ No

Completed by ________________ Date ________________

Questionnaire for gadolinium-based contrast media administration to be completed by the referring clinician

1. History of moderate or severe reaction to an MRI contrast medium	☐ Yes ☐ No
2. History of allergy requiring treatment	☐ Yes ☐ No
3. History of asthma	☐ Yes ☐ No
4. Does the patient have end-stage renal failure (eGFR < 30 ml/min/1.73 m^2) or is the patient on dialysis ?	☐ Yes ☐ No
5. Does the patient have reduced renal function[a] (eGFR between 30 and 60 ml/min/1.73 m^2)?	☐ Yes ☐ No

[a]Only necessary question, if high-risk NSF agents are used

Completed by ________________ Date ________________

Publications from the ESUR Contrast Media Safety Committee

Aspelin P, Stacul F, Thomsen HS, Morcos SK Molen AJvd, Members of Contrast Media Safety Committee of European Society of Urogenital Radiology (ESUR). Iodinated contrast media and blood interactions. Eur Radiol. 2006;16: 1041–9.

Bellin MF, Jakobsen JA, Tomassin I, Thomsen HS, Morcos SK, Members of the Contrast Media Safety Committee of the European Society of Urogenital Radiology. Contrast medium extravasation injury: guidelines for prevention and management. Eur Radiol. 2002;12:2807–12.

Bellin MF, Webb JAW, Molen AJvd, Thomsen HS, Morcos SK, Members of Contrast Media Safety Committee of European Society of Urogenital Radiology (ESUR). Safety of MR liver specific contrast media. Eur Radiol. 2005;15:1607–14.

Bellin MF, Stacul F, Webb JAW, Thomsen HS, Morcos S, Almén T, Aspelin P, Clement O, Heinz-Peer G, Reimer P, van der Molen A on behalf of the Contrast Media Safety Committee of the European Society of Uroradiology (ESUR). Late adverse reactions to intravascular iodine- based contrast media: an update. Eur Radiol. 2011;21:2305–10.

ESUR Contrast Media Safety Committee (Thomsen HS). ESUR guideline: gadolinium-based contrast media and nephrogenic systemic fibrosis. Eur Radiol. 2007;17:2692–6.

Jakobsen JA, Oyen R, Thomsen HS, Morcos SK, Members of Contrast Media Safety Committee of European Society of Urogenital Radiology (ESUR). Safety of ultrasound contrast agents. Eur Radiol. 2005;15:941–5.

Molen AJvd, Thomsen HS, Morcos SK, Members of Contrast Media Safety Committee of European Society of Urogenital Radiology (ESUR). Effect of iodinated contrast media on thyroid function in adults. Eur Radiol. 2004;14:902–6.

Morcos SK, Bellin MF, Thomsen HS, Almén T, Aspelin P, Heinz-Peer G, Jakobsen JA, Liss P, Oyen R, Stacul F, Van der Molen AJ, Webb JAW. Reducing the risk of iodine-based and MRI contrast media administration: recommendation for a questionnaire at the time of booking. Eur J Radiol. 2008;66:225–9.

Morcos SK, Thomsen HS, Exley CM, Members of Contrast Media Safety Committee of European Society of Urogenital Radiology (ESUR). Contrast media: interaction with other drugs and clinical tests. Eur Radiol. 2005;15:1463–8.

Morcos SK, Thomsen HS, Webb JAW, Members of Contrast Media Safety Committee of the European Society of Urogenital Radiology (ESUR). Contrast media induced nephrotoxicity: a consensus report. Eur Radiol. 1999;9:1602–13.

Morcos SK, Thomsen HS, Webb JAW, Members of Contrast Media Safety Committee of the European Society of Urogenital Radiology (ESUR). Prevention of generalized reactions to contrast media: a consensus report and guidelines. Eur Radiol. 2001;11:1720–8.

Morcos SK, Thomsen HS, Webb JAW, Members of the Contrast Media Safety Committee of European Society of Urogenital Radiology. Dialysis and contrast media. Eur Radiol. 2002;12:3026–30.

Stacul F, van der Molen AJ, Reimer P, Webb JAW, Thomsen HS, Morcos SK, Almén T, Aspelin P, Bellin MF, Clement O, Heinz-Peer G on behalf of the Contrast Media Safety Committee of the European Society of Urogenital Radiology. Contrast induced nephropathy: updated ESUR Contrast Media Safety Committee guidelines. Eur Radiol. 2011;21:2527–41.

Thomsen HS, editor. Contrast media. Safety issues and ESUR guidelines. 1st ed. Heidelberg: Springer; 2006.

Thomsen HS, Webb JAW, editors. Contrast media. Safety issues and ESUR guidelines. 2nd ed. Heidelberg: Springer; 2009.

Thomsen HS, Webb JAW, editors. Contrast media. Safety issues and ESUR guidelines. 3rd ed. Heidelberg: Springer; 2013.

Thomsen HS, Almén T, Morcos SK, Members of Contrast Media Safety Committee of European Society of Urogenital Radiology. Gadolinium- containing contrast media for radiographic examinations: a position paper. Eur Radiol. 2002;12:2600–5.

Thomsen HS, Morcos SK, Members of Contrast Media Safety Committee of the European Society of Urogenital Radiology (ESUR). Contrast media and metformin. Guidelines to diminish the risk of lactic acidosis in non-insulin dependent diabetics after administration of contrast media. Eur Radiol. 1999;9:738–40.

Thomsen HS, Morcos SK, Members of Contrast Media Safety Committee of European Society of Urogenital Radiology (ESUR). Management of acute adverse reactions to contrast media. Eur Radiol. 2004;14:476–81.

Thomsen HS, Morcos SK, Members of Contrast Media Safety Committee of European Society of Urogenital Radiology (ESUR). In which patients should serum-creatinine be measured before contrast medium administration? Eur Radiol. 2005;15:749–54.

Thomsen HS, Morcos SK, Almén T, Bellin MF, Bertolotto M, Bongartz G, Clement O, Leander P, Heinz-Peer G, Reimer P, Stacul F, Webb JAW, van der Molen A. Nephrogenic systemic fibrosis and gadolinium-based contrast media: updated ESUR Contrast Medium Safety Committee guidelines. Eur Radiol. 2013;23:307–18.

Webb JAW, Stacul F, Thomsen HS, Morcos SK, Members of the Contrast Media Safety Committee of the European Society of Urogenital Radiology (ESUR). Late adverse reactions to intravascular iodinated contrast media. Eur Radiol. 2003;13:181–4.

Webb JAW, Thomsen HS, Morcos SK, Members of Contrast Media Safety Committee of European Society of Urogenital Radiology (ESUR). The use of iodinated and gadolinium contrast media during pregnancy and lactation. Eur Radiol. 2005;15:1234–40.

Contrast Media Safety Committee Spring 2012
Henrik S. Thomsen (DK) *Chairman*,
Fulvio Stacul (IT) Secretary,
Torsten Almén (SE),
Marie-France Bellin (FR),
Michele Bertolotto (IT),
Georg Bongartz (CH),
Olivier Clement (FR),
Peter Leander (SE),
Gertraud Heinz-Peer (AT),
Sameh K. Morcos (UK),
Peter Reimer (DE),
Aart J. van der Molen (NL),
Judith AW Webb (UK)

Consultants
Eric Lancelot (Guerbet, FR),
Philipp Lengsfeld (Bayer Pharma, DE),
Alberto Spinazzi (Bracco, IT)

Appendix 2: Recommendations of European Medicines Agency for Minimization of Risks of Nephrogenic Systemic Fibrosis with Gadolinium Containing Contrast Agents

NSF

The EU Commission has approved the proposals from EMA regarding gadolinium-based contrast media.

ESUR Summary

Different measures to minimize risks have been taken for higher- and lower-risks GdCAs.

No differences have been made for medium- and low-risk products.

Measures Taken

Discontinuation of breastfeeding for at least 24 h is therefore recommended for all patients receiving high-NSF-risk GdCAs.

The use of high-risk GdCAs is contraindicated in patients with severe renal impairment. Strong warnings are included in the GdCAs of medium and low NSF risk as regards use in patients with severe renal impairment but subject to dose restriction to a minimum during a scan and with a minimum 7-day interval between administrations.

For patients with moderate renal impairment, since the risk is unknown for the high-risk category of GdCAs, it was agreed that use should only be considered after careful consideration of the benefit-risk, subject to dose restriction to not more than one injection of the minimum dose during a scan with a minimum 7-day interval between administrations.

Patients undergoing liver transplantation are at particular risk of NSF if exposed to GdCAs particularly to the high-risk GdCAs. Therefore, the use of high-risk GdCAs is contraindicated in this population. Strong warnings are included for medium- and low-NSF-risk GdCAs as regards use in this particular special population.

The use of the high-risk category of GdCAs in neonates up to 4 weeks of age is contraindicated. The use of medium- and low-risk GdCAs in neonates should only be considered after careful consideration, subject to dose and interval administration restrictions.

For all patients to whom high-NSF-risk GdCAs will be administered, mandatory screening for renal dysfunction by laboratory tests is required. This screening is recommended for all patients who will receive medium- and low-NSF-risk GdCAs.

Updated ESUR Contrast Medium Safety Committee guidelines on NSF see in the article "Nephrogenic systemic fibrosis and gadolinium-based contrast media: updated ESUR Contrast Medium Safety Committee guidelines". Euro Radiol. 2013;23(2):307–18.

Henrik S Thomsen, Sameh K Morcos, Torsten Almén, Marie-France Bellin, Michele Bertolotto, Georg Bongartz, Olivier Clement, Peter Leander, Gertraud Heinz-Peer, Peter Reimer, Fulvio Stacul, Aart van der Molen, Judith Aw Webb [less] Department of Diagnostic Radiology 54E2, Copenhagen University Hospital Herlev, Herlev Ringvej 75:2730, Herlev, Denmark. European Radiology (Impact Factor: 3.55). 08/2012; doi:10.1007/s00330-012-2597-9. Source: PubMed.

MIX
Papier aus verantwortungsvollen Quellen
Paper from responsible sources
FSC® C105338

If you have any concerns about our products,
you can contact us on
ProductSafety@springernature.com

In case Publisher is established outside the EU,
the EU authorized representative is:
Springer Nature Customer Service Center GmbH
Europaplatz 3, 69115 Heidelberg, Germany

Printed by Libri Plureos GmbH
in Hamburg, Germany